Gout Relief

Best Treatment Options to Relief Your Symptoms and Reclaim Your Life

(Step Relief Formula to Stop Pain from Gout Inflammation)

Allan Roberts

Published By **Zoe Lawson**

Allan Roberts

Gout Relief: Best Treatment Options to Relief Your Symptoms and Reclaim Your Life (Step Relief Formula to Stop Pain from Gout Inflammation)

ISBN   978-1-77485-994-0

No part of this guidebook shall be reproduced in any form without permission in writing from the publisher except in the case of brief quotations embodied in critical articles or reviews.

Legal & Disclaimer

Table Of Contents

Chapter 1: Introduction

In America, 8 million people had gout in 2003. These numbers indicate that pain affects 6% of the male population, and 2% in the female population. This disorder is more common in men than it is in women, as they have a higher blood uric content. After menopause, the disorder is more common in females.

The Latin word for "gutta," is a derivative. "Gout" literally means "a drop."

Gout was thought to be caused by toxic substances in the blood. This belief was common many centuries ago. This is not true. Gout is caused when there is an abnormal rise in levels of uricsäu in the bloodstream.

There are many questions when you are first diagnosed as having gout. Most people are unaware of what gout is and whether it can or cannot be treated. Gout can also impact your quality of life. It's common to have many questions after being diagnosed. They should all be asked.

This eBook is designed to provide the most basic information to help you understand your condition. This eBook will give you useful information about gout as well as treatment options. There will also be tips and suggestions on how to manage your gout so it doesn't have a negative impact on your everyday life.

We will be discussing the many options available for treatment. Many people depend on prescription medications to manage their gout. But there are natural remedies that can help. We will discuss the role of exercise in your condition and how it can be helped by changing your diet.

Gout is treatable. Gout isn't a life sentence. It is possible to manage your disorder effectively and live a happy and fulfilling life with the right knowledge. The outcome of any medical condition is dependent on your willingness to work hard and follow through with the treatment plan. All else will fall in place if everyone does their part.

Chapter 2: What Is Gout And How Can You Help?

Gout

Bone erosions

Urate crystals
in a tophus

Synovium

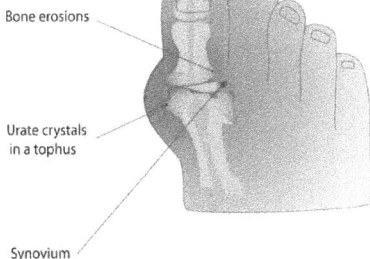

Gout, a blood disorder, is characterised by recurring episodes of inflammatory joint disease. "Podagra" is the name given to the attack on the bigtoe. Half of those cases involve the metatarsophalangeal joint or 'MTP' joint. It is most likely the bottom of your big thigh. Gout can also occur as kidney stones or acute urinary nephropathy.

You know by now that gout results from an abnormally high blood level of uric Acid. The uric acids crystallize and are released into the tendons and joints. Many tissues surrounding the affected area are also affected.

Gout has been increasing in prevalence over the past decade. Gout is estimated to affect around two out of every hundred people in the West. A rise in risk factors could be the reason for higher numbers. These factors include an increased body's energy and storage needs, a longer lifespan and changes in eating habits. Gout was known in the past as the "rich man's sickness".

Gout is a process that goes through four stages.

1 – Asymptomatic - Although the body has high levels of uric Acid, it does not show any other symptoms. This stage does not usually need treatment.

2 – Acute - This is the stage in which uric Acid crystals are deposited around your joints. Symptoms are usually experienced at night and last for three to ten consecutive days. A second attack may not occur for long periods.

However, attacks will not stop as fast as they get worse as time goes on.

3 - Interval: This is the period between acute attacks. During this interval time, symptoms are not present.

4 - Chronic: This is the stage that is disabling. The developmental phase can last over a decade. In this stage, irreparable damages can be done.

Chapter 3: Gout Causes

Purines are broken down in the body and made into uric acids. The body naturally produces purines. You can also find them in small fish such anchovies as herring. Gout has been linked with certain vegetables such as asparagus, mushrooms, and organ meats.

Uric acid can be dissolved and deposited through the kidneys into the urine. A buildup of uric, whether the body produces an excessive amount or the kidneys do not properly deposit it, can cause an imbalance in the body's ability to absorb the uric. This leads to needlelike urate crystalline formation. The crystals form in the joints and surrounding tissues. This causes pain, swelling and inflammation.

It is possible to develop gout in hyperuricemia, but many people who have it don't develop it. Hyperuricemia means that someone has a abnormally high level uric acid. Researchers aren't certain about the causes of hyperuricemia. The genetic factor has been established. It is more likely that someone who has hyperuricemia in their family will develop it.

Gout is one of the most common conditions.

1) Excessive alcohol intake. This is especially true with beer consumption.

2) A diet containing high amounts of purine.

3) This diet is very low in calories.

4) Use aspirin/niacin regularly.

5) Excessive drinking of drinks that have high fructose. Drinkers of these drinks are 75% more likely than women to get gout.

6) Rapid weight loss.

7) Chronic kidney disease.

8) Kelley-Seegmiller syndrome, Lesch-Nyhan syndrome.

9) Specific forms of anemia and lead poisoning

10) Surgery, the treatment of certain types of tumors, as well as some medications used to transplant patients.

More information will emerge about the causes of gout as researchers continue to carry out studies. Needless to mention, the list is expected to grow.

Who gets gout most often?

Anybody can develop this condition. However, gout is more common in males. Because of this, the female body eliminates uric acids more quickly. Gout can rarely occur in children.

These are just a few of the other factors.

** Age: Males between the ages of 40 and 50 are at greater risk for developing gout.

** Family history- Nearly 20% are related to someone with / who has gout.

** People who are overweight, obese, or suffer from obesity.

** High Purine Diets

** People with enzyme problems that cause the body to stop the breakdown of the uric Acid.

** Individuals who consume excessive alcohol

** Take Niacin and Diuretics as well as Salicylates

All of these are factors that contribute to the development of gout. Research is continuing to expand the list. These categories are important to consider when choosing a lifestyle.

Chapter 4: The Signs, And Symptoms

Gout can cause acute symptoms and signs that often start without warning. Most people notice the symptoms at night. They might feel severe joint pain in their feet, ankles as well as their wrists, wrists, and hands. This is a common problem area. It is common to feel a tightness in the joints from the inflammation of tissue. Olecranonbursitis can be caused by inflammation of the elbow. Prepalatellar bursitis occurs when the knee is affected.

One sign and symptoms can last more than seven days if left untreated. Over the next few days, signs and symptoms will slowly disappear. It is not uncommon for the itchy skin to begin peeling after the initial bout passes.

Reddening of the joints may cause swelling, tenderness and reddening. This is usually the place where the greatest pain is felt. The area may become discolored, with purple and red hues, which could indicate that it has an infection. Gout episodes can often cause high temperatures.

Joint inflammation causes limited movement.

You may feel less comfortable in your joints. Don't push your body too far. Nodules can be another sign and symptom that you may have gout. Nodules may first appear around the elbows and hands. While some people don't experience any symptoms, others end up with chronic or severe gout.

Check for gout

Gout can be diagnosed by two tests. After your physical examination, your doctor may decide to perform one or both these tests. A blood test can be used to check your blood for uric Acid levels. Because some people love to display symptoms, this test is often not conclusive. Some people with gout have normal blood levels of uric acid.

The joint fluid test is the second test. Fluid is drawn from the affected areas and examined for the presence of urate crystallines.

Chapter 5: Gout Treatment Options

Gout is treated with many medications. Your doctor can help you choose the right medication for you by looking at your symptoms and severity.

Corticosteroids is the most widely used medication. A corticosteroid could be prednisone. This medication is effective at treating inflammation and joint pain. Corticosteroids can lead to side effects like sodium retention, anxiety depression, depression, and the formation of ulcers. Long-term use can lead to more serious and permanent side effect.

Colchicines may also be an option. This is the most effective treatment if taken within 12 hours of the attack. This is a natural product, made from the "meadow-saffron" plant. There are small amounts of toxins in colchicines. However, the United States Food and Drug Administration declared it safe to use for the treatment of gout and other ailments.

The third treatment option is to use non-steroidal-anti-inflammatory drugs, or NSAIDs. These drugs can be used to treat inflammation when taken in high amounts. Aspirin, naproxen and ibuprofen are the most popular of this group. All these medications are available at your local pharmacy and can be purchased without a prescription.

As a preventive measure, some doctors may recommend certain medications in low doses. You may also be prescribed medications that lower your uric Acid levels.

Chapter 6: The Role And Benefits Of Your Diet, Gout Fighting Foods

Purines can be found in many of the foods we eat. You should know that the body converts purines into uric Acid when it breaks them down. You are increasing your body's uric Acid levels if your diet is high in purines. This can increase your chances of developing gout. This risk can also be increased by eating organ meats or certain seafood types.

Food

Limiting your intake of certain foods or beverages is a good way to limit the consumption of purines. These foods include:

** Meat

** Small fish (sardines or herring, for example)

** Gravy

** Beer

You shouldn't eat certain things. They aren't dangerous, even though they contain purine. These foods include:

** Fish and other seafood

** Wheat bran (and germ)

** Oatmeal

Reduce your intake of foods that may increase your risk of developing gout. The best way to manage your condition, is to change your diet. Your calorie and fat consumption may need to be monitored. You should increase your consumption of ow-fat dairy foods as they can help to reduce the signs and symptoms associated with gout.

Gout Fighting Foods

As there are certain foods that you should avoid, or eat in moderation; there are others that you should increase. The following foods can reduce uric Acid levels and help with pain and inflammation.

Bananas: High potassium levels in bananas help to convert urate crystals to liquid. They are then eliminated by the kidneys. The vitamin C content aids in pain management as well as inflammation. It is recommended that at least 2 bananas are consumed each day.

Cherries are rich in antioxidants. Cherry juice also contains anthocyanins which can prevent swelling and attacks. To reap the full benefits of cherries, it is recommended that you consume at least 20 cherries daily. Cherry juice mixed with minced garlic is another effective treatment.

Apples: Gout sufferers will know the value of an apple every day. After every meal, it is recommended that you have an apple. Apples are rich in malic acids, which help to regulate uric Acid levels. In turn, inflammation and pain are reduced. Similar results can also be obtained from carrot juice and apple cider.

Ginger root and turmeric both have healing properties that can boost your immune system and reduce inflammation. You can increase your garlic-turmeric intake by cooking with them. Also, garlic can be purchased in pill form. Cumin's curcumin can interfere with the signals that the blood vessels swell.

Pineapple: The high content of bromelain in pineapple makes it effective for treating inflammation associated with gout. It is believed the enzyme prevents the signal for swelling from reaching its destination. It helps to digest proteins which may lead to buildup of uric Acid.

Strawberries are rich in vitamin C, which helps neutralize uric Acid levels. The same is true for a wide range of grains and nuts.

Parsley, olive oil and eggs are other foods that can be used to fight gout. Also, you should add butternut squash and celery seed to your diet. You can find a wide variety of foods that fight gout. Keep it simple: Avoid food high in purines. Increase intake of foods high in antioxidants to reduce inflammation and neutralize uric Acid.

Chapter 7: Natural Remedies For Gout Treatment

There's a home remedy or natural way to treat almost any ailment. You only need to look. These treatments are easy and affordable for gout. You might find that many of the ingredients are already available in your own kitchen. If you've tried some of the remedies and they failed, you might want to think about how many times the treatment was tried. It might be worth giving it another chance, perhaps for a longer amount of time.

Cold Water: Cold water can be used to relieve swelling and pain. Use ice only on the affected area. It can make the situation worse. Allow the affected area to soak for 15 minutes every day. You can use an icepack up to twice per day. You shouldn't use an Icepack more than once a day as it can cause crystallization of the Uric Acid.

Lemon Juice can be used to neutralize blood uric Acid levels and alkalize the body. Make a mixture of the juice of one lemon and half a teaspoon of baking powder. Add it to a glass with water. Do not let the mixture sit. After mixing the ingredients, you should consume it immediately. You can also rebuild the tissues of your body with fruits high in vitamin C.

Baking soda: Baking soap has many uses. Baking soda is a great pain reliever and can help lower your levels of uric acid. The trick is to mix one-half of a teaspoon with a glass full of water. The mixture should not be drunk more than four days in a row. You can keep this mixture for up two weeks. Do not drink the mixture more than three days per day if your age is over 60. You should avoid this remedy if your blood pressure is high.

Epsom salt: Epsom salt can be used as a home remedy to many conditions, especially arthritis. Epsom salt's high magnesium content makes it extremely potent. The Epsom salt is a combination of warm water and Epsom sodium that can be used to relieve pain and inflammation. Once a week, add two cups Epsom salt to your tub. This should be done only three times per week if you are experiencing a severe attack. Allow your body to soak for as long as the water is still warm.

Activated Charcoal is able to absorb uric Acid. A charcoal bath twice or three times per week can help with inflammation and pain. Combine half a cup (or more) of charcoal powder with some water. Make a paste. Place the paste in a tub. Then, run the water. Allow your body to soak in the mixture for at least 60 mins. This natural remedy is great for treating gout. The paste can also applied directly to the skin, and left on for about half an hour. The paste can be removed with warm water. Also, you can take charcoal capsules in your mouth.

These natural remedies can relieve your gout pain and inflammation without side effects. You should remember that there is no immediate remedy. These natural remedies won't work immediately. They will be effective only if you use them regularly. Don't expect instant results. Check with your doctor to make sure these remedies do not interfere with your medication.

Chapter 8: Exercise And Gout

Gout can be controlled by exercising. It's common knowledge that exercise is important in the treatment of many forms of arthritis. By controlling your weight and blood circulation, adequate physical activity can reduce the amount of uric Acid in your blood. It reduces the chance of crystallized, uric acids getting into the joints. It is not unusual for pain to cause you to forget about exercise during an attack. A good amount of physical activity could be what you need to stop another one.

According to Mayo Clinic guidelines, excess fat and cholesterol may lead to the development of gout. Both can be reduced with exercise. Gout sufferers who are overweight or obese can ease the pressure on their joints and strengthen their muscles. The joint inflammation and pain can be decreased by placing less stress on it.

You run the risk that your joints become inflamed and cause you to move in certain ways. You should avoid exercising if you're experiencing flare-ups or other symptoms. If you experience a flare-up, it is important to rest your joints. Gout can be chronic. You rarely experience any symptoms. It is best to seek professional advice regarding exercise in order to prevent injury.

Your stage of gout, severity, and the joint conditions that are most affected should determine the types of exercises you choose. Gout sufferers often stick to low impact routines. Resistance exercises, swimming, walking and swimming are great ways to strengthen, tone and rebuild muscles.

Gout exercise

While gout may make you miserable, you can avoid exercising to prevent it from getting worse. It can make your condition worse and only make the symptoms you experience during an attack more severe. Joint pain can make you feel unwell when you move. You may experience joint pain and loss of flexibility.

Proper exercises can help control your gout, and aid in healing. You will experience a decrease or even complete elimination of your pain. You will notice an increase in energy levels, a decrease in weight and a better understanding of your joints, muscles, bones.

The following exercises will help reduce gouty symptoms. Strength training should include elastic bands to prevent injury. For preventing inflammation caused by improper form, smooth motions and proper form are important. You should exercise with a friend. This will ensure that if you do get in trouble, someone is there to help you.

Cardio and Aerobics

Cardio exercises improve the functionality of your lungs. They also increase your body's ability use oxygen to metabolize acid. Aerobic exercise is primarily intended to improve the strength of your lower-body muscles.

It is best to choose low-impact activities. For the first ten minutes of each exercise, you should do them every day. Gradually increase the time that you exercise each week. It is important to set a goal. The goal is to get 45 minutes of exercise per day. Allow yourself two days to rest. Low-impact exercise options include walking, swimming and the elliptical.

Swimming is a great way to improve mobility and function of joints. When you are in the water, gravity is not an issue. This eases some of your joint pressure. Similar to aerobic and cardio exercise, you should take it slow. You are only as good as your time when you exercise. Speed and distance don't really matter. Begin by swimming 15 minutes two times a week. Gradually increase your swimming time to 45 minutes per session.

Stretching is an excellent way to heal your joints. Spend some time every day moving your upper body joints by doing exercises that improve their range of motion. Here are some examples.

** For a minimum duration of 30 seconds, hold your hands straight at your sides. Roll your shoulder in one direction.

** Place your hand into a fist and then roll your wrist in each direction for at least 30 second.

It's important to also exercise your back, hamstrings and glutes. You can stretch your legs by laying down on the ground. Grab your toes, or reach for them. Hold this position for about 20 seconds. Repeat the exercise several times.

Mobility

There will be moments when you just want to get out of pain. This can lead to severe health issues. The crippling effects that immobility can have on your body is reduced by strengthening your muscles and joints. It doesn't necessarily mean you shouldn't take a quick walk. Keep moving around to avoid stiffening joints and muscles.

Chapter 9: Some Myths About Gout

Gout myths are a common topic that has been around since forever. If you do your research, you will find so many different stories that it can be hard to tell fact from fiction. It is disappointing that with so much information at our disposal, people remain so ignorant of the truth. Let's take a look at some of the myths about gout. Here are some common myths regarding gout.

Myth: Prescription drugs are not better than natural remedies

Colchicines are an effective natural treatment for gout. It is made from the plant meadowsaffron. This natural remedy is not toxic, but it is very effective. Many people who take high doses of these medications often experience nausea, vomiting, or diarrhea. A majority of these medications are prescribed to treat gout derived from natural sources. This does not necessarily mean that they are safe. These items are regulated and monitored daily by federal administrations.

This means they are safer than many natural alternatives available today. Vitamin C, for example can reduce uric Acid levels. However excessive vitamin C may lead to the formation of kidney stones. This could cause gout. If prescribed drugs aren't used properly, they can prove to be very dangerous. Even natural remedies can pose danger if they're not used correctly.

Myth: Gout medication works instantaneously

Low uric acids medications can actually cause flare-ups. It may take up to 12 months before they stop. If your medications don't stop working, the worst thing you can do is to stop taking them. An unexpected change in your levels of uric acid can lead to a flareup. Commonly, doctors don't prescribe the right dose of medication to lower your level of uric Acid. A lot of doctors also don't prescribe medications for prevention. At first, it may be best to begin with a low dose. You can gradually increase the dose over the next several days. Avoid stopping medication entirely. Instead, you should reduce the dosage over several days.

Myth: Every case can be treated with gout medication

Gout isn't a magical cure. There is no magic bullet. Gout is usually a result of something genetic. Gout can also be caused from other diseases. Gout can only ever be treated if the cause is genetic.

Myth: You'll stop eating seafood and drinking beer if you don't want to have gout.

When it comes to gout, the worst myths about diets is Diet Myths. Yet, many myths are true to a small extent. Consuming too much beer and seafood can lead to an increase in uric acid. It does not mean you will have fewer gout attacks if you stop drinking seafood and beer. These foods can be avoided to reduce your gout attacks.

Myth: Gout hurts, but it's not.

This myth is dangerous, and it is incorrect. Gout can be fatal if it isn't treated properly. Gout can cause severe damage to your joints if it is frequent and persistent. Tophus, which is an excessive amount of uric Acid crystals can lead to disfigurement. They can damage your heart and cause death if these crystals are present. Gout can be caused by excessive uric Acid in the bloodstream. High blood pressure, obesity and overweight are all contributing factors. All of these can cause death. Gout, although it may not look like a major threat to your life at first glance should be treated with seriousness.

Myth: Your weight is not an important factor in your gout.

You are wrong! Overweight and obesity have been shown to be linked with uric acid levels in the bloodstream. This is what causes gout. A healthy weight is the best thing you can do for gout management. Obesity and obesity are serious conditions. Gout is a serious condition that can lead to weight problems.

Myth: A terrorist attack is beyond your control.

It takes only 60 minutes to stop an attack if you take immediate action. This is dependent on the method you use to treat your condition. If you choose natural remedies, it may not work.

Myth: Science does not understand gout

Gout is one of most studied and understood diseases. Gout has been on the back burner of research since the 1980s. Gout has become a low priority, as almost 80% of doctors cannot properly treat the disorder. Gout management is a topic that has gained renewed attention, as it has in the recent past.

This is just a portion of the iceberg. You should seek out the help of someone knowledgeable about your condition if you are uncertain about anything related to gout. A rheumatologist (a doctor who is trained in the treatment of gout) is a specialist. Gout can be very serious, even though it may not seem like it.

Chapter 10: Gout And Depression

Gout can be a life-altering diagnosis Gout pain is not just physical. Pain can impact your mind, your actions and your disposition. Depressing pain is possible. Depression can make it worse. It's a "catch-22". The same chemicals are used in pain management as to regulate your mood.

Many with gout will confirm that the disorder can cause them to lose their ability to focus on other aspects of life. They don't want to be bothered, and they are not likely to be the most cheerful people. They focus on the pain and ignore everything else. Even the people who care the most.

Gout patients can feel stifled and lose their passion for life. Socializing may be the last thing on your list. It is important to be mindful of whether or not your relationships with loved ones are being eroded. It is common for gout to become more severe at night. It may happen because there is nothing else to distract you. It is difficult to focus when you are isolated.

There is a well-established association between depression, pain, and both. You can avoid depression by being able to identify the signs. Some of the symptoms include:

** Less energy

** Insomnia/excessive sleeping

** Changes in eating habits

** Feeling the "blues"

** Indifference to normal activities, including sex.

The process of dealing with any kind of health issue can be painful. To effectively treat your health condition, it is important to maintain a healthy mind. It is perfectly normal to feel low from time to another. It is important to not remain there.

Gout and its painful history

Gout has been around for many centuries. It has been documented in Egyptian mummies, which date back to 2640 B.C. Hippocrates, the first physician to attempt a description of what causes gout, was among the first to recognize it. (466-377 B.C.) For thousands of years, scientists have been trying to find a cure.

Gout is very painful and can cause severe pain.

Gout was common in the past, but t was mostly confined to the wealthy, such as the royalty and upper classes. Gout was thought be caused by obesity and alcohol overindulgence. It was only wealthy people who could afford such a lifestyle. Because obesity is becoming more widespread, the likelihood of it occurring is increasing.

Gout has been an issue for many famous people. King Henry VIII of England is the best-known case. Harry Kewell, an Australian soccer star, was diagnosed with the disease during his 2006 World Cup match. Maurice

Cheeks, a NBA player and Portland Trail Blazers coach, suffered his first gout attack in 1946. Jim Belushi is a well-known actor who has had gout problems for the past 15 year.

Gout can be treated with many different methods. Commonly, medications are prescribed. Many prefer the homeopathic approach. Other people use wives' tales to help with their gout. Some of these treatments are effective to some extent, but others are empty promises.

One thing is certain: gout can often be treated or even cured with a healthy diet. In addition to reducing sugars and refined grains, you can find relief. Although many diets include some of the recommended food choices, the Paleo lifestyle has been found to offer the best balance in nutrients as well as health building options. It offers a way to live a different lifestyle than our current one. Paleo is a diet that supports your body's functions. It also helps you avoid the triggers of gout attacks. It can help with many symptoms that you may already have, as well as prevent future attacks.

If you're looking for a permanent solution to the Gout pain and swelling, you should be familiar with the basics of the disease. This includes what causes it, how to get relief, and what you can do to prevent it from returning. You want to find out what works and doesn't.

This book was created with that goal in mind. I want you to be able to make an informed choice. My goal is to give you the ultimate solution to your gout. The solution to your pain lies in your control.

What is gout, exactly?

Gouty arthritis (also known as gouty joint disease) is a condition that causes painful inflammation in the joints. Gouty arthritis can be a very serious and recurring condition. It happens when your body is overloaded with uric acid.

Uric acid is formed when your body breaks down purines. These substances are found naturally in your body and in foods such organ meats as asparagus, mushrooms, and other vegetables. Both plants and animals have purines in their cells. They help to maintain the chemical structure of DNA and RNA. Normally, uric acids passes through the kidneys before it is excreted by the body as urine. Urate crystals can form either in the joints or around the area if the body produces too many uric acid or your kidneys fail in their duty to remove enough. This can cause inflammation and pain.

One person may only experience one attack of the condition, while others will have recurring episodes. One person can experience several attacks during a single year. People with gout can also develop kidney stones due to uric Acid crystals that build up in the urinary system.

You might also hear the term pseudogout. It can also be referred to as pseudogout. This is caused when crystals called calcium pyrophosphate accumulate around and in the joints. Pseudogout is similar to gout.

Pseudogout shares many similarities with true gout. However, pseudogout and gout have different appearances when the fluid that contains them is examined under a microscope. You can have pseudogout with gout.

How can I tell if this really is Gout

Gout attacks can occur suddenly, often at night and without warning. The most severe symptoms of gout include intense pain in the joints, especially in the big and middle toes. Red, tender, and swollen joints will indicate that they are affected. The skin around the joints is usually very hot. Some discomfort can last for several days or even weeks, even after the most severe pain is gone. If the pain recurs, it will usually last longer and affect more joints.

Gout can be diagnosed by a number of medical tests. A joint fluid test might be suggested by your doctor. He will use a needle and draw fluid from the affected joints. The fluid will be examined by a microscope to determine if there are urate crystallines. He might recommend a blood test which will check your blood for uric Acid.

What does gout look, exactly?

Gout is visible as a slight reddish swelling of the affected joint. However it can appear very serious and even grotesque.

What are the potential risk factors for gouty?

Some factors may contribute to high levels uric acid which can cause gout.

* Age / Sexe - Gout is more common for men than for women, and they are also more likely to develop it later in life.

* Heredity – It is more likely you will develop gout after your family members have experienced it.

* Lifestyle-Gout is caused by excessive alcohol intake, obesity, and sedentary lifestyles.

* Medical Conditions-If you have diabetes or arteriosclerosis, high cholesterol, high blood pressure or high levels fat and cholesterol you are more susceptible to developing gout.

* Medications: Anti-rejection medication prescribed for patients who have had organ transplants, diuretics to control hypertension, and low-dose aspirin can all contribute to the development gout.

What triggers a gout attack

Gout attacks can occur from a number of different factors. These can be combined or taken in isolation. It is best to avoid gout attacks if you are susceptible.

* A life that is overly stressed.

Consuming alcohol and high purine foods are the main causes of gout. These binges can result in rapid changes to blood uric Acid levels, which can be a trigger for gout.

* Cold is another. Avoid being outside in cold weather.

Gout flare-ups may also be triggered by heat and humidity.

* Some medications can cause hyperuricemia, which can lead to gout. This is most commonly caused by diuretics or immune system suppressors.

* Injuries such as kidney disease and heart disease.

* A joint that has suffered an injury in its past is more likely to suffer from gout.

* Infections

* Low dose aspirin can trigger gout.

* Environment factors such as lead exposure.

* The body's ability to excrete more uric Acid is dependent on how large it is. Gout can also be caused by obesity. It is possible to avoid becoming overweight or lose weight. This will help you feel better.

How can you help prevent future attacks

A 2012 research study found that a low-energy, low-calorie, low-carbohydrate diet (40% of energy), high quality protein (120g/day) with unsaturated oil (30% of calories) is more effective in lowering serum insulin, LDL, and triglyceride levels than the conventional low-purine diet .

There are some things you can do to lower the risk of having another attack. It is easy to make dietary adjustments that can significantly improve your chances of living with a gout-free life.

* Fluids- High fluid intake (with a high content of water) will help reduce uric Acid buildup and flush away toxins. Avoid sweetened drinks like soda. It is important to limit or avoid alcohol, including beer.

* Maintain your normal body weight. Avoid fasting or rapid weight reduction, which can temporarily raise uric Acid levels.

* Vitamins are helpful in controlling gout. Vitamin C and potassium Citrate can be

helpful in lowering uric Acid levels. Quercetin, an anti-inflammatory compound that helps relieve swelling and pain, has been shown to reduce inflammation. Chromium Picolinate is a great way to reduce obesity and lose weight. It also has positive effects on insulin levels. Pantothenic Acid has been shown to reduce uric levels. E Omega oils have anti-inflammatory properties and may decrease pain. Folic acid can be used to lower uric levels.

How common is gout?

Gout has been linked to increased blood pressure and obesity. Gout is more common among men than in women, with the risk increasing as you age. Gout accounts for about 5% in all cases of arthritis. Most people with gout are between the ages of 40-59. Gout can also develop in women. However, this usually happens after menopause. Gout is very rare in children and young adults. It affects more people than 8,000,000, or 4%.

Traditional treatment

Gout treatment includes the use of prescribed medication to reduce inflammation, swelling, pain killers and corticosteroids.

You may also be advised to modify your diet in order to avoid eating high levels of purines. Purines convert into uric Acid. Even though seafood and meats are low in purines, many doctors will still recommend that you follow a low-meat diet. Avoid foods such as liver, kidney, sweetbreads, organ meats, legumes (dried bean and peas), gravies, or mushrooms. The basic diet does not allow for animal protein intake. It recommends that you eat more plant-based, low-fat or non-fat dairy products and more grains. It also encourages the avoidance or limitation of alcohol consumption.

The Mayo Clinic is a world leader in medical research. They claim that strict dietary restrictions made it hard for gout sufferers to follow the diet. However, there are now less strict gout diets.

What are some of the most frequently used drugs for treatment?

Some medications have been used for the treatment of acute attacks and to prevent future attacks.

Nonsteroidal Anti-Inflammatory Drugs (NSAIDs), which include Advil Motrin Motrin, Advil, Motrin and Aleve, are effective in controlling inflammation and pain in people suffering from gout. A higher dose may be required to treat an acute attack. However, a lower daily dose is necessary to prevent future attacks. These drugs, especially those that are used for long periods, may cause stomach pain, bleeding, or ulcers.

Colchicines may be prescribed to those who are unable use NSAIDs. However side effects can include nausea and vomiting as well as diarrhea. A doctor may prescribe you a low daily dose colchicine to treat acute gout attacks.

Corticosteroid medicines can be used to control gout inflammation. Prednisone is one such medication. These medications are available in both pill and injectable forms. Corticosteroids can only be used in patients who can't tolerate NSAIDs, or colchicine. Corticosteroids could cause severe side effects like thinning bones, slower healing and reduced ability to fight infection. Most physicians will prescribe the lowest possible dose of these drugs to manage side effects.

If you have severe pain or suffer from multiple gout attacks throughout the year, your doctor may recommend medication.

Allopurinol (or febuxostat) can reduce the body's uric acid levels and decrease the likelihood of more attacks. Probenecid works by lowering uric Acid levels and improving kidney function. Probenecid can cause stomach pain, kidney damage, rash, and skin irritations.

New drugs are used to treat

Researchers are constantly trying to bring new medicines on the market that treat a condition more effectively and with fewer side effects. This is true for both gouty and other diseases.

The long wait for a new drug to treat gout was not over. Uloric, the FDA's first drug to treat gout, was approved by Takeda Pharmaceuticals. It reduces uric Acid production and lowers elevated uric Acid levels when taken orally every day.

Pegloticase (which converts urine into a chemical compound that's more soluble in blood) is another drug currently awaiting FDA approval. This drug worked well in patients who were exhausted by other therapies. Pegloticase maintained a steady level of uric Acid throughout the study. It was tested in patients and showed that it could regulate their uric levels in just six hours. The most common adverse reactions were joint pains, anemia headaches, joint pains, joint swellings, fever, muscle spasms and nausea. The researchers deemed the majority "mild" or moderately severe.

What about side effects of the drug?

There are many side effects to drugs that can lead to serious and unwanted side effect, especially when they are used with other drugs. These side effects may not be experienced by everyone who takes a drug. However, it is important that you read all information about your prescription so you know what to look out for.

Long-term use of NSAIDs has been linked to stomach pain, bleeding, or ulcers. Colchicines can cause nausea, vomiting, diarrhea and other side effects.

Uloric can have a number of side effects. Although rare, they do occur. These are just a few of the possible side effects.

* abdominal pain, stomach fullness, or discomfort

*arm, back, jaw, or stomach pain

* Chest pain/intenseness

* diarrhea

* hard or labored breathing

* dizziness

* fever

* Increased heart rate

* nausea and vomiting

*

Prednisone could cause the following side effects:

* Agony

* Anxiety

* blurred sight

* dizziness

* Headache

* irritability

* mental depression

* Weight gain

There are some side effects that Allopurinol may cause in some people. These are:

* Agony

* bruising

* chest pain/intenseness

* Chills

* Confusion

* constipation

* Cough or hoarseness

* Swallowing blood

* difficulty breathing

* dizziness

* Drozing

What are the homeopathic remedies tc gout

When you find out you have gout, you need to be able to see the problem from both a long-term and a regular perspective. It is also important to address both the symptoms and the underlying cause.

Gout is a condition that has been treated by homeopathic remedies for many decades. They are based on the belief of the body being capable of healing itself. Homeopathic medicine functions in the same way as vaccines or flu shots. One is given a small amount of the same substance causing the symptoms and it can be used to treat the illness. This means that the body's self-regulatory and normal healing processes are enhanced with a small dose of the same substance.

These medications are available in either liquid or pill forms and can contain small amounts of active ingredients (usually a herb or mineral) to treat disease.

Gout treatment by homeopathy involves treating the entire body. It does not treat symptoms. The homeopathic remedies do not cause harm to the body. They have no side effect. There are many homeopathic remedies to treat gout.

Arnica has been used to alleviate the pain associated with gout for many years. It is available in a variety of forms, including a pill, tincture and gel. The gel can be applied externally to provide maximum relief.

Belladona provides fast relief for swelling and pain. It is especially helpful when the joint is extremely sensitive and sensitive due to high temperatures.

* Berberis vulgaris is good for pains in the gouty joint or when walking or changing your position causes pain.

Calcera Fluorica should be used when severe pain is present and the joint is visible to swelling. It provides immediate relief.

* Rhus Toxicodendron treats sudden pains and swelling. It's useful for all types, including rheumatoid.

* Sulphur can be used to treat itchiness and pain in the joints. It reduces swelling and pain. This may affect the knees as well as other joints.

Homeopathiv Remedies can also be used to relieve the severe attack-related pain, stiffness, swelling, or discomfort.

Home remedies that can be used

Gout can be treated with natural remedies and home remedies. They are safe to be used along with conventional medications and treatment. Deep-breathing exercises and mediation are great for pain relief. Certain foods have been shown by research to reduce uric Acid levels. They are especially helpful in preventing attacks from returning. Some of these include, among others:

* Coffee – The powerful antioxidant, called chlorogenic acid, found in coffee may help to improve insulin sensitivity in individuals who are insulin resistant - which is a common

cause of gout. Coffee's xanthines, and/or antioxidants, inhibit uric Acid production.

* Vitamin C - Vitamin C is a good supplement to help lower your uric Acid levels. However, it's not as effective as prescriptions.

* Cherries- Cherries have flavonoids called Anthocyanidins. These can block pain and lower levels of uric.

* Blackberries: Blackberries are high antioxidants. Their alkalizing effects on your tissues can reduce the symptoms associated with gout. Blackberries have been used for centuries as a natural cure for gout. Flavonoids, which can be strong antioxidants, are high in protective nutrients.

Blueberries - Anti-inflammatory foods such as blueberries can reduce inflammation. Blueberries contain potassium, which helps to reduce inflammation and uric acid.

Cinnamon mixed with honey in boiling hot water for tea has been shown to be effective in the treatment of arthritis and other conditions like gout. One-third of the participants experienced a decrease in their symptoms within a week or a month. Nearly all reported significantly greater mobility and far less pain.

Flaxseed oil can be used to treat many diseases of the respiratory system, eyes, throat, joints, arthritis, and even gout. Many people with gout claim that flaxseed oils have helped to alleviate their pain.

* Lime: The citric Acid found in lime helps dissolve excess uric acid. Vitamin C found in lime helps heal sore joints, and strengthens tissues. To see visible results, you should drink half of a lime's juice in a glass of water every day.

* Pineapple has the most natural bromelain. The fruit is well-known for its ability to decrease swelling, redness and bruising. Bromelain causes uric Acid crystals to dissolve, which helps relieve the pain associated gout.

* Purple Grapes – Purple grapes, together with other potassium-rich fruits, have been shown in studies to reduce the symptoms of rheumatoid and prevent painful gout attacks. Recently, it was discovered that grapes can help prevent gout by lowering the blood levels.

Here are some other natural remedies to help you feel better.

Pain relief can be achieved by applying a paste made from charcoal powder and water to the affected or swollen area. Take 30 minutes to soak in this mixture.

Ginger root, devil's root root, white willow root, boswellia (boswellia), feverfew and licorice all have anti-inflammatory qualities that may reduce the symptoms associated with gout.

Baking soda (bicarbonate or soda) is another home remedy. It has been used for decades. This an old favourite remedy that many people who suffer from gout swear by. This is supposed to elevate your pH level, and even relieve or end your symptoms of gout. It usually works quickly, which is the good news.

Safflower can reduce the pain and inflammation associated with gout by increasing blood circulation.

Warm water mixed with ground ginger is a good way to get rid of uric acids.

Are home remedies effective?

Gout prevention is as important as gout treatment. Good food choices and a healthy lifestyle are key to keeping uric levels down. Gout attacks are usually caused by foods. These home remedies are proven effective and have stood up to the test of time. Combining them with diet changes can improve your health and help prevent gout attacks. Although they won't eliminate all symptoms, they may make the attacks less severe and more manageable.

Finding the best home remedies

These home remedies have been proven effective over the years. These are the remedies that our grandparents used. They couldn't run to the pharmacy or doctor as quickly as they used to. They used products that were available at their homes or in close proximity. Medical science was able to offer new solutions, so the old ways fell out of fashion. Many of the traditional methods produce better results. They can also be used to supplement modern medication for the best results.

* Ice has been used throughout the history of mankind to reduce pain and inflammation. The application of ice directly on the affected area works today just as well as it did in the past.

* Aspirin (or ibuprofen) will ease your pain.

* It is important to exercise your joints in order to prevent injury and reduce pain.

* Epsom Salt and hot water are good options for treating affected joints. Epsom salts

contains Magnesium. Magnesium can be increased to improve circulation and heart health. It can flush out heavy metals and toxins from your body. Warming your feet in Epsom Salts will provide almost instant relief from gout symptoms.

* Fresh strawberries are good for neutralizing uric Acid, as are nuts, seeds, and grain.

* Cherries are an old remedy for reducing uric acids.

* It is important to drink plenty of water to flush out toxins, and dilute uric Acid levels.

* Inflammation can be reduced by eating fruits such as tomatoes, citrus fruits, green peppers, and leaves.

Apple Cider Vinegar, one of the most effective home remedies, is one of its best. Gout pain can be reduced by 2 tbsp organic apple cider Vinegar mixed with 2 tablespoons Organic Honey taken twice daily.

Why the Paleo Diet might be the ultimate cure

Paleo lifestyle follows the same diet as our ancestors: Paleo includes animal foods, vegetables, fruits and nuts in season. t was often called the "caveman" lifestyle, as it used foods that cavemen, who were hunters, gatherers, and farmers, relied upon. It was a natural diet and beneficial for their natural health. It is possible to change your diet and prevent gout by eating a healthier diet.

The Paleo Diet has been shown to have positive effects on heart disease and nerve issues, as well as diabetes. It is common to have both diabetes and gout. Metabolic syndrome and insulin resistance lower kidney function, making it less efficient for the kidneys to remove uric from the body. The Paleo Diet helps reduce insulin resistance and metabolic syndrome as well as diabetes. This, in turn, lowers the amount in your body.

Conventional medical wisdom suggests avoiding low-fat dairy foods, as they can increase insulin resistance. It is better to avoid meat, as it actually reduces insulin resistance. Paleo has been shown far to be a superior choice.

What is the Paleo Diet, and what are its benefits?

Our diet is heavy on processed food and sugars. We consume fast food and sweets like cookies, cakes, ice cream, and donuts. And we drink lots of soft drinks. These modern health issues include obesity, diabetes, and heart diseases. If we eat a more natural diet, our bodies are healthier, stronger and more energetic.

Paleo is a diet based on the foods our ancestors consumed. We don't want to imitate the caveman with this diet. Instead, we are trying to adapt it for our current food choices. We will use our ancestral history to guide us in reclaiming our bodies, health, and lives.

The Paleo diet recommends that we avoid toxic foods.

Grains

Legumes

Vegetable seed oils

Sugar added to sodas, candies and cakes as well as fruit juices.

Sources of milk high in protein and sugar (lactose), as well as low in healthy, butter-fat.

Paleo means to eat nutrient rich foods.

A vast variety of vegetables are available, including root, starchy, meats, fish, seafood, healthy oils, eggs, fruits, nuts, and seeds.

Leafy green vegetables (spinach, kale, swiss chard, arugula)

Meat from grassfed ruminants (beef/bison, lamb)

Mollusks, oysters, mussels, wild Salmon, and sardines are all examples of Mollusks

Egg yolks

Bone broth

Fermented foods like sauerkraut and kimchi

Paleo living and eating habits promote a strong immune system and body that is resilient to infection. Paleo approved foods can be found online in an extensive list. You can find a great example here. http://ultimatepaleoguide.com/paleo-diet-food-list/

Paleo is easy to follow. It doesn't require you to track calories or keep track of what you eat. It's tasty, nutritious, and can greatly improve your health. It can reduce body fat, improve your digestion, and help with chronic pain. It can eliminate the risk factors associated with gout. This makes it the best gout solution.

New scientific research reveals what causes gout.

Gout has been associated with obesity, overindulgence and drinking. Obesity is associated with insulin resistance. This causes high triglycerides. high blood pressure. diabetes, stroke, chronic kidney disease, heart attacks, elevated uric acids, and increased triglycerides. Gout seems to be more common in people who are obese.

Modern research shows a strong connection between the development of gout, fructose consumption, and especially soft drink intake. We now know that the metabolism of fructose plays a significant role in the formation of uric acid. Fructose, an increasingly popular form of carbohydrate, has been shown in human studies to raise uric acid.

A person's carbohydrates intake will determine how much weight they have. The more a person weighs, they will consume more carbohydrates. Many scientists believe that gout is caused by an excess of fructose and carbohydrate in the diet. Excessive fructose consumption is the main cause of obesity and gout, especially central obesity. You can convert some fructose into uric Acid if you consume more than 25g per day. The bottom line is that high fructose syrup and sugar are likely to cause chronic toxins. It is important to eliminate them from all your diets, especially if they are causing obesity.

There are many common foods and ingredients that contain fructose.

* Fruit

* Fructose

* Corn Syrup

* High Fructose Corn Syrup (HFCS).

* Sucrose

* Table Sugar

* Sugar Cane

* Beets

* Cane Juice

Rice Syrup

* Maple Syrup

* Agave Nectar

* Fruit juices or nectars

* Soda Pop

* Who Are At Risk From Gout?

*

* Gout is a form or arthritis. It can be very painful. It is caused by the buildup of too much uric acid in your joints. You may be wondering what uric is, the dreaded devil that builds up in your joints and causes such intense pain. The pain is not caused by acid, as horrible as it sounds. It is actually the crystals that are formed from uric Acid buildup. Each person is affected by uric and susceptible to crystals forming. It is essentially a waste product. The body usually passes it through the kidneys as purines are released from cells that die. This includes purines the body absorbs from food we eat.

Hyperuricemia refers to excessive uric Acid buildup.

* You can easily trigger an attack by just taking a walk, or even banging your big toe against something. High purine foods or alchohol intake can also cause an attack. When you have had foot surgery, make sure you do not move your foot until it is completely healed.

* Who are at risk?

* The simple answer is that everyone is at-risk, but most people are walking a lot and eating certain foods in excess. We'll get to those later in this report. Some lifestyle choices are more likely to make you vulnerable.

* Lifestyle choices that contribute to your well-being

* Drinking excessive amounts of alcohol has been shown to raise the risk factor.

*

* Untreated Conditions

* Medications may also increase the risk. Some medications are required, such anti-rejection drugs that are prescribed for organ transplant recipients. Hypertension medication can also increase the risk. Low dose aspirin can be used to prevent heart attacks and strokes. But, it may also increase your chance of getting gout.

It can be frustrating to try to cure one thing, but it could also cause more problems. You need to decide what is the best choice for you.

* Other Contributing Factors

* Family History - This will help you determine if your risk is through heredity.

*

* Your gender and your age. Women generally have less uric acid than men. Although men are more susceptible to gout

than women, they tend to develop it earlier than the women.

* Frequency of Gout Attacks

* Gout attacks may occur in different ways for each person. You are not all the same.

* What is gout?

* You may experience uric Acid crystals in your kidneys, which can lead to a painful condition called uritide crystals.

* Now that you have a basic understanding of the disease and its symptoms, as well as the risk factors and reasons for it, you can start to look at diet and treatments for the symptoms of gout.

* Reduce or eliminate high-purine foods from your diet to prevent gout. As we stated earlier, purines are responsible for uric Acid production and buildup. It is caused by heavy red meat and fish eating. This is frustrating because many people try to change from meat to seafood to improve their health. But

this is a serious condition that can be treated by changing your diet. If you are overweight, then you might consider a slower weight loss plan. But, it is important not to lose too much weight, as this could cause you to have an episode.

*

*

* The Best Natural Cure to Gout

*

* We'll go through the diet first. It is important to follow this diet if you want to be able to use natural cures.

*

* Meats and fish high in purines

* Herring

* Mackerel

* Anchovies

* Tuna

71

* Red meat is composed of beef and lamb

* Pork

*

* Other foods to be avoided

* Fatty dairy products

* Avoid sugar

* Foods to Eat When You Have Gout

Keep hydrated

* Eat complex carbohydrates

* Gout sufferers often turn to natural remedies

* Vitamin C can be combined with other remedies for the gout.

Gout treatment can also include vitamin B12 (a common vitamin for energy).

* Drinking a few cups of cherries every day or a pound a day can help reduce the pain of gout. However you will need to be a big

cherry lover and have the financial means to afford it.

* Uric acid levels will be lower by drinking milk and yogurt at least one time every other days

* Bananas

* Strawberry's, blueberry's

* Celery

* Tomatoes

* Green leafy vegetation (e.g. cabbage, kale)

* Bromelaine rich foods

* Chocolate!

* Coffee and tea

* Seeds

* Tofu

* This list gives you an excellent selection of foods that can be carried around.

*

*

*

*

*

*

*

* Anti-inflammatory foods

* This special list is provided because the basis of natural medicine in any form of arthritis is inflammation. Doctors will give you (NSAIDS), which can be non-steroidal and used to treat inflammation. Prescription anti-inflammatory medication may contain steroids. This can be dangerous, as steroids may cause other issues or mood swings.

* When taken in sufficient quantities on a daily bases, the over-the counter version can prove to be dangerous. You can get liver and stomach issues, as well as a slower metabolism that could lead to more attacks. But, you'll get a better, safer result if you add anti-inflammatory ingredients.

* A little bit about natural remedies

* Before we dive into more lists you dive into drinking and eating pounds of this stuff per hour, because naturally, you are in pain. Before you start, I'd like to share some facts.

* Organic medicine is the core of every synthetic medicine. This means that all medication in your medicine box is made of natural herbs. Even if you use the herb to treat a condition, it may still be necessary for you to take it in a limited amount of time per day. It can also affect other medications you take. This is particularly true when you take blood thinners. Do your research and use common sense when you administer herbal remedies to yourself. Some of these remedies may cause adverse reactions.

*

*

* Now, let's look at the natural anti-inflammatory options:

* Ginger root

* Cactus & cactus juice

* Seaweeds & Kelp

* Turmeric

* Wild salmon

* Shitake mushrooms

* Green tea

* Papaya

* Blueberry's

* Extra virgin Olive Oil

* Broccoli

* Sweet potato

*

* Cactus or cactus juice is the most effective anti-inflammatory food. It is possible to order

liquid form online under several company names. It has been proven very efficient and effective with no reported adverse reactions. Green tea is great at reducing inflammation. You should drink 4 to 5 cups of it per day. Ginger root can also help with other inflammation and pain that can cause disorders like premenstrual syndromes and menstrual cramps.

* What is the best way to prevent gout attacks?

* First, we can review the five main methods to prevent a attack of gout. Then we will discuss what to do to relieve it. This is because it is essential to understand this information so we can avoid gout attacks.

* Recap:

* Lose weight

Keep hydrated

* Avoid high purine foods

* Check out the list of fruits and veggies

* Regular exercise

Weight loss is important because it is the most common factor in gout. This will make it much easier as you'll lose weight by drinking water, exercising, and eating fruit and vegetables. When you give up sugar and sweets, it will increase your metabolism. It will also regulate blood sugar.

* The gout is a blessing in disguise. If you want to be healthy and slim, it may be. The pain associated with gout will encourage you to change your lifestyle.

* What can you do for relief if you have an attack?

* While we will be interested in gout, and your diet as it has been described several times in the report, As we mentioned at the beginning, losing too much weight can lead to a flare up. We understand that the process of moving from a painful and difficult gout life to a pain-free gout life (because there is no cure) can sometimes be difficult.

* What remedies are available to treat gout flare-up? These common denominators are important to remember at every stage of the process.

* Water: It is the oil running the machine that is your entire body. This cycle is repeated because inflammation cannot be cured without it. It pushes hormones, chemicals and blood through the body into the joints. It also regulates metabolism. This is the root cause of gout.

*

* Ice compresses Applying cold ice to the affected areas will provide an external solution. You have several options. It is crucial that you don't burn already sensitive skin.

*

*

* Place the ice in a bag or cover it with a washcloth.

*

* The ice is applied in a couple of minutes and then taken off.

* Heating the area. This is a contradictory statement, but some people claim that it can provide relief. There are also cold and hot sports rubs. You can also place the rice in an uncooked sock, then heat it in the microwave. This will keep the heat in the microwave for several hours. The time spent in the microwave can vary so you should experiment. There are herbal packs that can be used for cold or hot compresses. The instructions for how to use them are included. They are basically herbs that can smell amazing and encourage relaxation when heated.

*

* Diet short-term. We discussed earlier the long-term effects on gout resulting from diet. There are foods and beverages that will work after you have started the regimen. One option is ginger root. This can be used in foods like stir-frys, but it is also great to boil

hot water for tea throughout the day. The ginger root can also be used in green tea. This gives it an interesting flavor and a combination of honey and cherries makes for a powerful anti-inflammatory food trio. The juice of cherry or at least one pound per day of cherries will work within the first 24 hours.

*

*

* Anti-inflammatory medicines: The last resort should be anti-inflammatory medication that can be prescribed or over-the counter. But as we mentioned earlier, it can take quite a bit to find relief which could be dangerous for your organs.

* These are some of the best ways to get rid of an attack quickly and with minimal injury to the body.

* I Am In Constant Pain. Is there anything I could do to change it?

*

* Chronic pain can be debilitating and severe. This society has many conditions and diseases that can be caused by stress, food or other factors.

* What does that have do with gout symptoms? The cause of chronic pain for many people is swelling. This holds true for chronic pain in any part. It is because of this that a lot is the same treatment. So how do you treat chronic pain? As we said earlier, the solution cannot be found at the root cause of the pain. This is the most common mistake made in diagnosing and treating these and other conditions. This is the mistake that both patients and doctors make. It is only a bandaid to cover a wound.

*

* If you have chronic pain, it is crucial to find out what is causing it before you try to treat the symptoms. A diet is often the cause, especially for swelling-based chronic arthritis. There are many things you need to know before you begin any treatment.

82

* There are many disciplines that we can discuss. We will cover diet again, and you should follow it strictly in all the disciplines covered in this section.

*

* The Pantry Must Have The Following Foods And Diets To Avoid Constant Pain

*

*

*

*

*

*

*

*

* If you're suffering from chronic pain, it is important to create a lifestyle around the treatment. Lifestyle changes are essential to help you form healthy habits that will be

carried on throughout your life. This is a printable workbook you can use to help you follow your new lifestyle. You won't be distracted by all the details of your new routines and lifestyle changes.

* Purge the junk in your pantry to cure chronic pain. This is how we start. When you begin to eat in a healthy way, you will soon be pain-free.

* Pantry purging. Below is the list. While we understand that change can be hard, we will provide an explanation. Some of it will be quite self-explanatory. Remember that there are food banks available if you are concerned about the waste.

* White sugar

* White Flower

* White Potatoes

* White rice

* Sugar

* White Refined Sucralose

* Salt

* Any canned or boxed food

* Fruit juice containing fructose corn sugar

* Corn Syrup

*We will begin with these. It seems that we are trying to cut off your life of fun and food, even though it is quite long. When you stop eating foods that make you retain water, it can actually make your condition worse. You must ensure you aren't retaining water if you have a condition like this.

* To replace the previous list, here is a list.

* Fresh fruits & vegetables

* Brown or raw sugar is acceptable if it is necessary

* Kosher Sea Salt Only if You Must

* Not from concentrate

* If you feel the need, make your own juice

* Whole grain breads/cereals

* Pineapple and Cantaloupe

* These are not the only basics, but it will rid the body of any bad food that could cause uric Acid to build up and spread to the joints. It is actually the blocking the source of the uric acid, and not a bandaid that will cover up a wound.

* Stop stress and let your body release natural pain killer hormones like dopamine and serotonin. Yoga is one option. This is great for conditions uric acid-based.

* Yoga will allow the muscles to be stretched in a way that releases uric and also lactic acid. You can also make food changes to reduce the amount of lactic acids that build up in your muscles, which will worsen the gout condition. It is also responsible for other conditions, including RLS (restless-leg syndrome) and other forms. It is an unrelated condition to gout and can cause it to worsen.

* If you're not quite fit enough to do traditional Hatha or Namaste Yoga, Bikram Yoga will be a better choice. Bikram Yoga uses dry heat. We recommend that you bring a towel, plenty of water, and plenty of food to ensure that you don't become dehydrated. This can cause counterproductive effects.

* Meditation is an excellent addition to Yoga. Stress is the main cause of chronic pain in arthritis. Research is showing that stress is a key factor in chronic pain. When it is controlled, it can be reduced.

* Chronic Pain Clinics

* Pain clinics are for those who prefer a more traditional approach. These clinics are new and growing all over the country. These clinics are covered under most insurance. They can train your brain and body how to eliminate and deal with pain.

* Alternative Methods

* NLP may also be an option if you are open to other methods. NLP is Neuro Linguistic

Programming. This is a similar method to hypnosis. Although it is technically hypnosis, it has been recognized as a better method by the medical world. NLP changes the brain's thinking. It can be used for anything, from business success to pain and many other things.

* The first appointment is to assess the situation. Next, you'll be brought into the alpha state. This is the Alpha state of your brainwaves. It is the state before sleep. If you're in this state, you can make suggestions to change the way that your brain receives pain impulses. It can actually stop nerve impulses from reaching the brain. It is usually associated to a touch or action, which is repeated when the suggestion is made to reinforce it.

* For instance, you might convince yourself that the sky's purple and not blue. After you have made your initial suggestion, and you are in Alpha brainwave mode, you will now suggest that you will know that the sky's

purple when you touch your right foot with your left arm. This can also be done with other people by touching the shoulder or arm of another person and repeating the suggestion. This is because your subconscious will respond more strongly to subtle, straightforward actions and words than your conscious.

* Acupuncture/Acupressure

* This is another popular and effective method to eliminate chronic pain that can be caused by arthritis. This is because the body and its line energy are responsible for controlling everything, from weight gain and cravings to metabolic disorders like hypothyroidism. Gout sufferers have good news, as it is a metabolic condition. It will also help to disperse uric Acid and prevent it reforming.

This can be done by placing sterile needles beneath the skin, and then opening the meridians. These are the energy centers within the body. This will help ensure that energy or chi is distributed properly and that bottled-up acids are released.

*

* Tracking of your progress

Journaling your progress is a simple way to keep on track as you try out these new methods. You will be able to see if you are making progress with each method. It can be time-consuming and expensive to use too many methods that don't work. This is, however, a way of determining if you are doing well with particular methods or a combination. This helps you choose which methods to stop or which ones to continue.

* On the next page, you'll find the questions required to correctly chart.

Chapter 11: Gout: What Is It?

Two issues are important to understand if you have gout. 1) How to stop an existing attack and 2) How can you manage your condition and prevent future attacks. You should consult a doctor if you are experiencing gout attacks. The faster you seek treatment, the less severe the condition will be. Some gout sufferers swear by injections of painkillers/anti-inflammatory agents straight into the affected joint, but oral medication is more common. Gout attacks should not be treated with aspirin unless you have been advised by your doctor. It could make the condition worse. Avoid alcohol, sugary soft drink and vitamin C pills. Some people, not all, believe that cherries can be eaten, or they can drink cherry concentrate (without sugar) and pop cherry pills. Drinking coffee is okay, but it's important to stay hydrated. Take your joint to the top of your heart, and take away any shoes/clothes that could stress it. You can ice the joint up to 15 minutes once per day. You shouldn't do too much. Rest. You should also see a physician to receive your medication. This book will help you learn how to prevent future gout attacks by recommending diet and medication.

What is gout, exactly?

Gouty arthritis, commonly known as "gout", is a painful and debilitating form of inflammatory arthritis that affects approximately 1-2% of adults in developed economies. Monosodium Urate crystals build up in or around joints, other tissues, and can cause inflammation and pain. Gout can be treated when serum uric Acid concentrations fall below the monosodium urine saturation point. The Greek "arthro", which is a Greek word meaning joint, gave rise to the term arthritis. Gout comes from an old European word for "droplet" or "drop", which is gote, gotta and gutta. Gout was thought to be caused from "disease" that drops into and onto the affected joints[2]. The truth is even stranger.

Gout is an age-old disease. Researchers have found evidence from bone samples that suggests that Tyrannosaurs Rex was affected by gout. Hippocrates[3] is the persor who first described gout. He lived in fifth century BC. He linked gout and lifestyle, which is a view that most people still hold to this day. This explanation may have merit, but it does not tell the whole story.

The attack

Anyone who has suffered an acute attack of gout knows what the word "painful" means. You may not have heard of "painful" but anyone who has experienced an acute attack of gout knows what that means. Like the illustration above, crystals resemble small toothpicks. Gout attacks usually occur at night, and can wake you up in the morning. Research suggests the reasons could be due to lower body temperatures and dehydration that favor precipitation (solidification?) of uric Acid[4].

It is important to note that adequate hydration (or drinking enough water) is an important factor in managing gout. We'll discuss it later. Gout sufferers may be able to control their condition by simply drinking enough water.

Uric Acid crystals can buildup and deposit anywhere within the musculoskeletal. Gout flares are usually limited to one joint, with 80-90% of cases[5]. Usually the lower limbs are affected, with most cases affecting one of the big feet (metatarsophalangeal Joint). The podagra is the name given to a gout flare. Gout tends to deposit uric acid in joints that have been damaged previously. Gout attack is most common in the 40- to 60-year-old age group. Gout typically develops in women following menopause. Some people believe that patients with gout may have enzymic problems if they develop it before the age of 25,[6].

You may experience severe pain from an acute gout attack. Long term gout can also lead to permanent damage to your joints. Tophi is a condition that forms around the affected joints. However, don't be fooled by the fact that your gout may have been diagnosed in recent years. Tophi may develop early in the disease. Gout isn't something to be taken lightly.

Gout can be caused by several factors

Gout is commonly referred to as a joke disease. However, many people see it as a painful and harmless disease that can be caused by eating too much and drinking too much. But is this true or false? How can gout develop? What are the other health issues and diseases linked to gouty?

Some things we are quite familiar with, others we only assume. If urate concentrations (or levels of uric acid) exceed their solubility limit at 6.8mg/dL at 37 degree Celsius, the substance solidifies and forms crystals within tissues. Gout sufferers must be familiar with hyperuricemia. This refers to excessive y high levels in blood uric acids. It is usually at 6 mg/dL (or higher) for women and 6.8 for men. But numbers may vary depending upon the laboratory.

Gout risk increases when there is high uric Acid levels. Gout incidence per year is 0.1% among patients with uric Acid levels below 7 mg/dL. 0.5% is between 7-8.9 mg/dL. 4.9% are over 9 mg/dL. [8]

So controlling gout involves at least partially controlling uric Acid levels.

But, not everyone with hyperuricemia will develop it. Gout incidences are "just" 22% for patients with a urate level of 9mg/dL. Scientists don't understand why patients with hyperuricemia do not develop the condition. Additionally, people who experience an acute attack can have low levels of uric Acid. Uric acid levels are very important but difficult to understand.

Hyperuricemia can cause gout. It is caused by excessive uric Acid levels. Even if your blood uric level is normal, crystal formation will occur if there is a high amount of uric Acid in the blood. While high levels over time are necessary to prevent gout from developing, it doesn't necessarily mean that you will get gout.

How is uric acid made?

Uric acid, also known by its name "weak acid", results from the metabolic breakdown and metabolism of purines. It is often referred to as a waste product of purine metabolic. Purine, one of the two kinds of nitrogenous bases that make up the basic structure of DNA or RNA, is also known as purine. Put another way, purines can be found everywhere you eat. You might have heard purines can cause gout. But all foods contain them. You don't have to avoid purines. It is absurd. However, gout sufferers should be cautious about eating foods high in purines.

Purines can also be found in high levels in the internal organs of the kidneys, livers, and brains. Sweetbreads, brains, beer and herring are other rich sources. All these foods are rich in purine. Moderate sources include meats and poultry, fish, seafood, poultry, and seafood. Vegetables and legumes like spinach, asparagus, mushrooms, and spinach are also considered moderate sources. Is it possible that meat consumption could cause gout? Perhaps not, as meat is a moderately rich source of purines.

Gout can be reduced by consuming purine-rich food. This is the "tip", which most gout sufferers repeat over and again. It is true that only about 30% of blood's uric Acid content is due to diet. Even if purines are a problem, diet will only reduce it by 30%. However, 30% could be a tipping point that can help those suffering from gout. I believe that controlling your diet could help you beat the gout. What do you need to know about diet? Is it enough to cut back on purine-rich food? What foods are restricted for gout patients? How do purines cause "goutal damage"? Are all purines bad. Are there other foods to be cautious about? Are there foods that can manage or prevent gouty? We will be discussing both the classic answers and the more recent studies. Over the past ten years there have been many new ideas and inputs.

We'll also examine dietary tips that may help prevent gout attacks.

Are you an over-excitor?

It is also important to know which mechanisms are responsible for your "gout". One reason gout sufferers might have high levels is because they either overproduce uric (this could be due to eating too much purine rich foods or a problem metabolizing purine), or (2) the uric o does not leave enough. The main cause of hyperuricemia (80 to 90%) is inability of kidneys to excrete the uric Acid. It is possible to lower the amount of uric, by decreasing your intake of purine rich food or other dietary modalities, but this will not make a big difference in terms of gout.

Gout can increase your risk of developing other diseases such as diabetes and heart disease.

Gout is an important condition. You need to be aware that it is a serious disease. Gout and other illnesses can often co-occur or become apparent over time. "Metabolic syndrome" is something to watch out for. This includes a variety of health issues, such as abdominal obesity and hypertension, as well as abnormal lipid levels and insulin resistance. It is important to note that hyperuricemia is a part of the metabolic condition. Patients with gout are more likely than those without it.

In patients with high cardiovascular disease risk, hyperuricemia increases cardiovascular mortality. So clearly, gout is more than "inconvenient" and dangerous. Gout sufferers have nearly twice the risk of dying from a heart attack, stroke, or both[10].

More examples of how gout can cause other problems Gout is a sign that you may be at increased risk for type 2 diabetes. Persons with high levels uric Acid can also get kidney stones. All of this is a sign that you must control hyperuricemia or gout. Not only is it a source of arthritic discomfort and pain, but also because of the other diseases associated with it.

Too much uric Acid

Let's review briefly. Gout is a chronic illness that is associated long-lasting high levels of uric Acid in the blood. Hyperuricemia can also occur, although a flare up or an attack of gout may not be caused by high uric level. Hyperuricemia can be defined as the highest blood urate concentration above the MSU (monosodium urine) solubility limit. This is 6.8 mg/dL for 37 degrees Celsius. Hyperuricemia in a relative sense is when MSU concentrations exceed the upper limit for the "normal" range. For men, this is 7 mg/dL, and for women it is 6 mg/dL. It is high levels of urine acid that cause crystal buildup, but it may not be the case for all. There are two possible causes of high levels: overproduction or under-excretion.

Uric acid, which is produced by the liver, is secreted into [1]the blood. Two thirds of the uric acid, or about two-thirds, is then secreted by the kidney into the urine. You then urinate it. The remainder is distributed through saliva, gastric secretions, and bowel. The uric, which didn't disappear through the normal channels, simply remains in blood. It may cause problems like gout. Many cases of hyperuricemia result not from eating too many purine-rich foods, but from impaired renal excretion. The kidney is not producing enough uric Acid through the urine. You're an "under-excretor".

Gout Attacks

Gout may occur after years of accumulation of uric Acid crystals in the joints, and the tissues surrounding. Even though a gout attack can often occur suddenly, it is more common for patients to feel mild pain in the affected joints. An attack that is severe can be prevented by being treated immediately. The pain often occurs at night and can be very painful. The pain may be intense and sometimes described as "being on Fire" in the affected joints. This can cause redness, swelling, and inflammation in one or more joints, including the big toe. Gout can also affect multiple joints at once.

Moderate attacks can last from a few hours to a couple of days. The soreness can last upto one month and severe gout attacks may last up to two days. Most patients experience a second episode of gout within six to two years. However, attacks can occur at different times. If gout is not treated, the likelihood of having attacks increases.

Gout has traditionally been divided into three to four stages by doctors. Research has shown that chronic gout is easier to diagnose and treat.

The stage of asymptomatic hyperuricemia

Gout can be diagnosed at any stage, but the first stage is one without symptoms. Because gout is always associated with high uric Acid levels, it's called asymptomatic hypouricemia. This is the initial phase of high levels of uric acid. There are no symptoms so most people don't even realize they are there. However, a blood sample will show an increase in uric acid. This initial phase can be slow. It can take years for the MSU (monosodium, urate) crystals to form. These crystals do not appear in all people. Signs and symptoms are only common in around a third of these patients. These are the people who get gout. The rest of the population will not experience gout. Asymptomatic hyperuricemia, however, has been associated with other disorders such as hypertension and chronic kidney disease. It is not a good sign to have high levels of uric Acid.

Acute gouty arthritis

Gout symptoms are the first stage. The second stage is characterised by the formation crystals in the joint. This is called acute, or gouty arthritis. After an attack, the symptoms will diminish and time passes. It could take many years. Attacks can then re-occur again and resolve. There is less time before the next attack and so forth. The interval between attacks could be shorter.

Gout attacks may become more severe or last longer in later years.

Before the first full-blown attack, there may be smaller attacks of less intense pain in the affected joint. This could happen years before the actual attack. It is not necessary to be extremely sensitive to recognize that you are experiencing gouty, painful arthritis. This is the time when the pain starts. It is rare for more than one joint to be affected by the first attack. If left untreated, the attack will peak in 48 hours and cease after a week. This could be shorter or longer. The acute gouty joint can be treated, but there are not many reasons.

Intercritical gout, chronic tophaceous Gout

The intercritical period is when there are no attacks. Normally, the symptoms and signs of gout disappear after the first attack. You may have tophi if you have already had multiple attacks. Depending on the severity and extent of your problem you may reach the fourth stage chronic tophaceous Gout.

Under the skin may develop tophi-like nodules or sandy nodules. Tophi can form in the cartilage of your outer ear and the surrounding tissues (tendons, ligaments or bursae) if you don't get proper medical care. If left untreated, patients can suffer from severe bone and cartilage damage.

Older people may experience the stage 4 symptoms more quickly.

Chapter 12: Risk Factors And Their Causes

Primary gout means that gout can occur by itself without the presence of any other diseases or conditions. Secondary gout can occur when gout comes with another condition or disease, or is caused due to certain medications or procedures. Primary gout cases make up 99% of the cases. The reasons for high uric Acid levels are not understood. The reason for high levels of uric acid is not known. However, genetics and hormones could play a role in this.

Gender and Age

There are certain things that we know. These two indicators are age and gender. Gout is more common in males than in females. Could this be partly due hormones? We know that uric Acid levels rise dramatically during adolescence. But, age also matters. It is more common in men older than 30 years. Could it be that this disease has been accumulating over the past decade and a-half since puberty? It is just waiting for some people to reach tipping points at the 30s. Maybe it's because of diet. Could be. If so, it would prove very helpful to test young men for uric Acid levels in their 20s. This will allow them to be treated early if they are in danger. We know that women are less susceptible. It is uncommon for women to experience this condition until after menopause. Hormones may also play an important part in this condition. Premenopausal women are at a lower risk of developing it than men. This may be because estrogen levels in the blood facilitate the release and kidney function of uric Acid. Only 15% of cases of gout in women are before menopause. After menopause, the risk of developing gout increases for women. Gout can be diagnosed in both men and women at 60 and 80. It is more common in women than it is among men.

Obesity

Gout prefers men. This is because it is associated with high levels of cholesterol, high bloodpressure and unhealthy eating.

Gout and obesity are strongly connected. You can control your weight to prevent gout and reduce the severity of gout. Research shows that 71% are overweight, according to some studies. The risk of developing Gout in 21-year old men is twice if they are overweight. Individuals who have lost 10 lbs or more reduced their chance of developing gout by 30% (Choi, 2005). Research has shown a direct link between bodyweight and uric Acid levels. One Japanese study found that obese people are more susceptible to hyperuricemia (up to three times higher) than those who have a healthy weight. As a result, children who are overweight will be more susceptible to developing gout.

Obesity, in and of itself, is a risk factor to other diseases such high blood pressure, cardiovascular disease, and so on. Gout sufferers also have to be aware of the risks. Obese gout patients are more likely to experience gout-related complications than those who aren't obese.

Gout genetics

You are more likely to be diagnosed with gout if your parents have it. Research has shown that 20% of all gout sufferers have a family history. A few people who have a family history with gout have deficient enzymes which affect how the body breaks down purine. Although genetics play an important role in the development gout, your family might also have the same habits as you. Gout is often linked to excessive drinking of alcohol. The risk of developing gout in children born to heavy drinkers is higher than for those who don't.

Gout medications that are likely to cause or worsen gout

Gout can also be caused when you take certain medications. Gout is most commonly caused by thiazide-diuretics (water pills). These water pills are used to reduce excess salt and water in the body. Talk to your doctor before you start diuretics. If you don't feel the need to switch to other blood pressure medications, your doctor may recommend medication that lowers your body's production of urine acid such as allopurinol and febuxostat.

Low doses common aspirin may reduce the body's ability get rid of uric Acid. This is a common reason for taking aspirin. You may be able to switch to other drugs to prevent strokes or heart attacks. Patients who have had an organ transplant are frequently given anti-rejection medications. This can make them more susceptible to developing gout. Gout could also be affected if you take pyrazinamide and Niacin.

Alcohol

Gout can be caused by alcohol. Not only does it increase uric acid production but it also reduces the body's ability remove it. Gout is most commonly associated with beer. This is due to the presence of guanosine which is a purine. The risk of getting gout from mild wine drinking is not increased. Gout is strongly linked to alcohol consumption among young adults. Binge drinking raises body levels of the uric acid. The role of alcohol in older patients, especially those with gout, appears to be minimal.

Dieting

Gout can also be caused by diets that are protein-based, extreme or fasting. Fasting can trigger gout due to an increase in body ketones (alkanones).

Dehydration

This is likely a little-known and poorly understood aspect of what could trigger gout in people with gout. According to my own experience, hydration may have a strong impact on the prevention and/or reduction of gout attacks. Gout sufferers, however, need to be more aware of the importance of water intake and hydration. While it is well-known that good hydration is important, many people struggle to drink the required 3 liters of fluids per day for men and 2.2 liters daily for women. Specialists believe dehydration can cause an increase in blood levels of uric acid and even a gout attack. For more information on diet, please refer to the chapter.

Organ transplantation

Transplantation of kidneys can raise the risk of gout and cause renal insufficiency. Gout may also occur after other transplants like liver and heart. Gout can result from both the procedure (cyclosporine), and the medication taken by transplant patients (leukemia). Gout can also result from treatment for other diseases, such as psoriasis (leukemia) and psoriasis (psoriasis).

Other medical conditions or lead poisoning

The effects of treating other medical conditions could cause an increase in blood uric acids, which can trigger a Gout attack. These conditions include lymphoma or leukemia and psoriasis. A high incidence of gout and the development of uric Acid is associated with occupational exposure to lead.

Chapter 13: Diagnosing The Condition And Testing

Sometimes, gout can be hidden or mistakenly interpreted as another condition. However, most people do not require a test to determine if they have gout. Gout usually shows up in the second stage, which is when symptoms begin to appear. Most people can identify gout symptoms such as joint pain and swelling. The doctor might simply say that you have an attack. This is only the start of your journey. It is important to take tests.

Gout can only be confirmed by performing a joint fluid analysis (arthrocentesis). To determine if there are uric Acid crystals at the joint,

For gout diagnosis, you will need to get a blood test. It is however, a strong indicator. The blood test should include white blood cells, WBCs as well as triglyceride (high density lipoprotein), glucose, kidney and liver function tests. For those with high blood uric levels, a 24-hour urinary acid evaluation will be necessary to determine the ability of your kidneys to eliminate it. Unless you have advanced gout, Xrays may not prove helpful. There are other imaging tests that may be required depending on your individual situation. This is usually the case for advanced stages.

Blood test for uric acids

No prerequisites are required to pass the test. The test results may be affected by certain medicines. Be sure to inform your doctor about any medication, prescription or not. A nurse or healthcare practitioner will draw blood from the vein on your arm during the test. The majority of lab results list reference values, which can vary depending upon the laboratory. The range of values must be stated in the laboratory result. Your doctor will review the results and make recommendations based on your medical history. You might find that the result is not as normal as the ones listed below.

The normal uric levels for children are 1.0 to 5.5 milligrams/deciliter (mg/dL), or from 119 to 237 mmoles/liter. Normal uric acid levels for men range from 3.4 mg/dL to 7.0 mg/dL. This is 202 to 416 micromoles per liter (coml./L/). Normal uric acid levels for women are 2.4 to 6.0 mg/dL.

Joint fluid (synovial fluid) analysis

Synovial fluid (or joint fluid) is typically a thick, straw-colored liquid found in the joints. The fluid acts as both a lubricant in the joint and a cushioning agent for the joint. It is necessary to take a sample of the liquid with a needle. This sample will be sent to an analysis. The sample will be tested visually for color as well as under a microscope for crystals. The test will count the number of red blood cells and white blood cell, as well uric acid measurements. You don't usually need to be prepared for the test and it takes only a few minutes.

Chapter 14: Treatment

It's hard to imagine someone with acute gout symptoms not wanting to take medication to relieve inflammation and pain. Gout treatment typically involves the use commercial drugs. Although they may be effective in treating an acute attack, there are also over-the counter medications such as Advil and Aleve. While some may argue that these over-the counter drugs for gout do not work, they can be helpful if they are taken promptly at the onset and/or just before the attack. This is when you will feel some pain in the affected area.

Gout treatment can include drugs that may be helpful in long term management.

Many people think that long-term use of gout medications can be dangerous. People may be scared of taking potent drugs for long periods of time, or because they have gastrointestinal issues and/or heart problems. They try to avoid gout drugs and believe they can beat it with a change in their diet, lifestyle and avoiding certain foods. This is a personal decision that will depend on your beliefs. These choices depend on the severity and type of your gout. You can beat gout by changing your lifestyle and eating right. Don't underestimate the risks of high uric acids levels. You can keep an eye on your levels and take steps that will keep them down.

Your medical history and preferences will play a role in the prescriptions you receive. Some medications interact with other drugs in a strong way. Your doctor might recommend a different drug.

It is important to treat

Gout medicine is used to treat acute attacks as well as preventive attacks. This usually involves addressing the causes of high uric Acid levels. While it is obvious that you need to take medication for acute attacks, this doesn't mean you should ignore the underlying causes. If it isn't treated, it can lead to serious problems such as the formation of tophi (from urate crystals).

Hyperuricemia can also lead other diseases. It is important to maintain a low level of uric acid.

You need pain relief and antiinflammatory medication when you have acute gout attacks. You must address your high uric Acid levels once the attack has ended.

Gout attacks in the acute phase

An array of anti-inflammatory substances can be used to treat an acute gout attack. They include colchicine (NSAIDs), glucocorticoids(GCs) as well as nonsteroidal antiinflammatory drug (NSAIDs), colchicine (GCs), and, more recently, interleukin-1, (IL-1), inhibitors like Canakinumab or Ilaris. Studies have shown that NSAIDs as well as low-dose collchicine, GC and canakinumab all work to treat acute gout. However there isn't enough evidence to rank them. It is quite expensive, and might be a good option for those who are unable or unwilling to use NSAIDs. A 150mg dose is approximately USD $ 18,000.

A doctor should be consulted as there are many factors that could affect the safety and effectiveness of your drug, including any other conditions you may have or drugs you are currently taking. Particular caution is needed if you have impaired renal function, gastrointestinal issues or cardiovascular problems. A doctor must decide which medication you will use.

It is important to get anti-inflammatory medication started as soon as possible after the attack. Rapid treatment can reduce the severity and duration of the attack. It also helps to speed up the recovery process. The amount of medication that you need to take may be reduced if you are quick to treat. Your medication would normally last five to seven working days if it is started within 12 to36 hours after symptoms first began. You should start treatment no later than 12 hours.

You will normally need to take a higher dose at the beginning. If symptoms begin to decrease, you can reduce this dose. The treatment should be continued for several days after the attack is over. These are the medications that can be used to treat acute attacks of gout and prevent future attacks:

Non-steroidal Antiinflammatory Drugs (NSAIDs),

NSAIDs decrease swelling, fever, or pain. There are many NSAIDs to be used for acute gout attacks. NSAIDs can be used for acute gout attacks in patients younger than 65, as well as patients without any medical problems.

You can subdivide NSAIDs in two main groups. In order to relieve pain and treat inflammation, NSAIDS used two enzymes: COX-1 & COX-2. Newer NSAIDs focus on COX-2 enzymes. These NSAIDs have the added advantage of not causing stomach problems, bleeding, or obstruction. This is because COX-1 protects the stomach lining and these newer NSAIDs are also called COX-2 antagonists. COX-2 does its job. COX-2 is a better option for patients with stomach issues and those who started their gout treatments late [12]. Although there are side effects that have been reported, including cardiovascular problems, many COX-2 drugs have been withdrawn from the marketplace over the past decade, most notably Vioxx. Although the scientific evidence is not conclusive [regarding cardiovascular safety of COX-2 inhibitions], it is widely believed that COX-2 prevents a protective hormone (which can dilate arteries in cases of cholesterol buildup) from leading to strokes. Celecoxib is the COX-2 inhibitor NSAID most commonly used in treating gout. Indomethacin and naproxen (Aleve), as well as sulindac and Clinoril, are the most common NSAIDs used for gout.

Side effects are common with all drugs. Many warnings are given about NSAIDs. This is because they are a very potent class of drugs. Although some medications are available over the counter, it does not mean that they don't pose risks. NSAIDs can cause kidney damage, especially in the elderly or in patients with already existing kidney disease. Most doctors will tell anyone with kidney disease to stay away from NSAIDs. This is true even if there are peptic ulcer diseases or anticoagulation therapy.

Side-effects most commonly caused by NSAIDs include heartburn, stomach upset and stomach pain. Long-term use is more likely to cause stomach ulcers, bleeding, high blood pressure, allergic reactions, such as hives, asthma, face swelling, hives, and asthma. There are many other NSAID medications, and every one is unique. Some NSAIDs may increase the risk for stroke, myocardial ischemia, and cardiovascular thrombotic episodes, but these risks can be small with short-term treatments[14].

Avoid NSAIDs if: You are 60+, pregnant, consume more than 3 drinks per day, have a kidney disease, liver problem, take blood thinners or take medicine to lower your blood pressure. Talk to your doctor if there are any concerns about high blood pressure and/or if you take aspirin to protect your heart health, such as preventing strokes or heart attack, before you start taking any other NSAIDs. You should consult your doctor immediately if your gout is related to your heart condition. Low doses may increase uric Acid levels and can cause flare ups[15].

OTC NSAIDs can be purchased over-the-counter (OTC). These include low dose ibuprofen ("Advil, Nuprin"), ketoprofen ("Actron"), naproxen sodium ("Aleve"), and aspirin ("Bayer), Bufferin," Excedrin). You can get stronger doses of these drugs by obtaining a prescription. Prescription NSAIDs can include celecoxib, Motrin, and Indomethacin (Indocin). The individual's response to gout may vary depending on their condition. If NSAIDs are indicated, doctors could prescribe 800mg of ibuprofen or 25-50 mg of indomethacin, three to four times per day.

Corticosteroids

You can choose not to take NSAIDs if you don't want to or if it is impossible for you to do so, corticosteroids are an alternative (prednisone). These powerful drugs can stop inflammation and reduce pain. Your doctor can inject cortisone intraarticular (only if one joint is involved in a gout attack). The cortisone may be administered orally to any other joints that are being affected. Pills are another way to put it. Some patients swear by injections as soon as they feel the onset of a severe gout attack.

Corticosteroids are generally prescribed to patients who aren't recommended to take NSAIDs and colchicine, patients with severe gout, or for patients with gout attacks involving more than one joint. Although corticosteroids have been shown to work as well NSAIDs, studies suggest that they could be used more frequently for gout [16]. Doctors usually recommend a dosage of 0.5mg of corticosteroids, or prednisone, per kg. Once daily, body weight until flares weaken, on full dosage for 2 to 5 days. Taper

126

off for 7 to 10, then taper off for 5 to 10, then full dose for 5-10, and then stop.

Warnings come with corticosteroids such as prednisone. The drug lowers the immune system, and can increase infection risk. It mimics your body's natural cortisol hormonal response. Corticosteroids could cause cortisol to be less effective if used for too long. There may be side effects such as high blood pressure, fluid retention or mood swings. Patients with bacterial arthritis should not use corticosteroids. High blood pressure should be monitored during corticosteroids treatment. Diabetes patients may need insulin and more medication when receiving corticosteroids to treat gout.

Colchicine

Colchicine, one of the most well-known gout drugs, can be prescribed by your doctor. Colchicine is used in both acute and long-term treatment of gout. However, it doesn't reduce uric Acid levels. It is not clear exactly how colchicine functions. It acts as a "mitotic inhibitor" and terminates cell growth. Additionally, it binds with proteins in the microtubules and white blood cells of neutrophils and reduces pain and swelling. It has no effect either on uric Acid production or excretion, but reduces the inflammation reaction to urate stones. However, colchicine does have some anti-inflammatory effects, however, it is not as effective in treating other inflammatory diseases like gout.

It has a very narrow therapeutic index which means that the difference in a toxic dose and a therapeutic dosage is very small. As with any drug, colchicine can be administered intravenously orally as well as by injection. However, serious toxicities are associated with intravenous colchicine. Oral administration of colchicine is the preferred option. Doses as low at 7 mg have been shown to cause fatalities. Please note that grapefruit juice could increase the risk of colchicine poisoning.

Acute gout attacks can be treated with colchicine. If you're already taking colchicine prophylactically but are suffering from a gout attack and have not had any gout flares in the last two weeks, your doctor may ask you whether you used high doses of colchicine. This is a reason to use colchicine. Gout treatment used to be as simple as 1.2 mg colchicine for initial symptoms, then 0.6 mg per hour for six-hours or until symptoms subside or you get diarrhea or stomach problems, which can indicate early signs of toxicity. Colchicine toxicity and recent studies that prove low-dosage colchicine treatment works have led to a general recommendation for lower doses and longer intervals [18]. Today, the recommended dosage is 1.2 mg colchicine in the beginning and 0.6 mg after an hour. These may be just as effective and have less side effects. However, it is best to stop using colchicine immediately if you feel any abdominal pain, nausea, vomiting, diarrhea, or burning sensations on your stomach, throat, or skin. This is a typical recommendation. Patients with hepatic impairment, elderly patients (above 60), and those who are overweight or obese will be advised not to take any other medications. This decision is entirely up to your doctor.

After an intensive colchicine regimen, your doctor may prescribe one-tablet-a day. You should wait at least a few days before recommending another intensive regimen. Your doctor may suggest a lower dose for future attacks, depending on the severity of your acute gout.

Colchicine has been around since long. Colchicine, a plant-based alkaloid, was first extracted from the Colchicum Family of Plants (autumn and meadow saffron, Gloriosa superba, and glory lilly). Colchicine is used to treat rheumatism. We also have Egyptian papyrus descriptions. There are texts dating back to the first century AD that provide details on the treatment of gout.

Interactions of other drugs: Are there any calcium channel blockers (diltiazem), macrolide antibiotics(erythromycin), antifungals/fluconazole), certain antifungals(fluconazole), PGP inhibitions (clarithromycin), clarithromycin and erythromycin? These drugs could increase your risk of colchicine toxicity [19]. Although your doctor will know exactly what is best for each patient, they will most likely recommend that you reduce the amount of colchicine you take or to avoid toxic effects. Patients with severe renal or liver impairments may need to be advised not to take colchicine. Colchicine may cause men to lose their fertility[20].

Colchicine toxicities symptoms: These include abdominal pains, vomiting, nausea, diarrhea, and nausea. These symptoms could be signs of intoxication from colchicine. These symptoms could include hypotension or electrolyte imbalance. Delay symptoms may include seizures and cardiac dysrhythmias, hypotension and shock, coagulopathy and pancytopenia.

Chronic Gout Treatment/ULT Therapies

Other than colchicine, medication to treat acute gout is different from medications to prevent gout from escalating.

Gout prevention medications include uric-acid inhibitors and uricosurics.

* Uricosurics (probenecid)

* Allopurinol is an inhibitor of urac acids

* Enzyme converters

* Mitotic inhibitions (colchicine).

Gout sufferers have to lower their levels of uric. However, there are many ways to achieve this. The right drug for you depends on your situation. It also depends on any other illnesses you may have or other medications you take that could interact with gout drugs.

* Uricosurics - helps excretion

* Inhibitors - diminishes production

* Converters-Uric acid conversion to harmless byproducts

* Colchicine-unknown action

There may be a problem with your excretion. In order to assist with the excretion uric acid, certain uricosuric drugs (probenecid and benzbromarone) target specific mechanisms in your kidneys. Are you overproducing your uric acid levels? The best option is to use inhibitors like allopurinol (or febuxostat). Let's take an in-depth look at these treatments.

Uricosurics

These drugs, which include the well-known and widely used probenecid, which is next to allopurinol or colchicine, are meant to improve the elimination rate of uric Acid. They do not reduce or stop the production. If the patient is suffering from moderate gout and has not had any previous kidney complications or developed kidney stones, uricosurics might be indicated.

Uricosurics are kidney specialists who direct uric in to the blood, increase excretion of urine (as opposed the blood), and lower blood uric acid. 20% of gout sufferers have gout because of under-excretion or even partial uric acid deficiency. Treatment with uricosurics is possible for those who are suffering from gout.

By taking a 24-hour urine testing, you can determine if there is an underexcitability of uric acids. Interpreting these results to determine whether you are underexcreting uric Acid is up to your doctor. There are many opinions about where the limits should be set. There is a risk that you could start to secrete too many uric acids, which can lead to kidney stone formation. This should always be a concern.

Drink plenty of fluids to reduce the risk of kidney stones. Gout sufferers will need to drink more water. Talk to your doctor about how to fix your urine if it is too acidic. The best thing to do is to take sodium bicarbonate. But this is not recommended for people who have to monitor their sodium intake.

A prescription for Uricosurics is not available to people over 60. The best thing is to make sure your kidneys are healthy before starting uricosurics. These drugs can also have contraindications so be sure to check this information and inform your doctor if you are taking any type of drug.

There are several types of uricosuric medications: Primary uricosurics drugs drugs are drugs where the drug's primary effect is its uricosuric one. Primary uricosurics: Probenecid (Benemid, Probalan), sulfinpyrazone; isobromindione and atorvastatine. Secondary uricosurics: Losartan, fenofibrate (Guaifenesin), amlodipine (atorvastatine), fenofibrate and fenofibrate. Probenecid (Benemid (Probalan), the uricosuric drug that is most commonly used to treat gout is Probenecid (Beremid), together with sulfinpyrazone.

Benzobromarone (a stronger uricosuric) is not recommended for patients with severe gout (tophaceus, or severe tophi). The other uricosurics can be used in some cases. Benzobromarone could cause liver failure and is not permitted in the US without a special authorization. One study demonstrated that benzomromarone is even more effective that the XO-inhibitor, allopurinol. That will be reviewed shortly. Some studies question the safety of this drug being removed from certain markets [22].

The effectiveness of the uricosurics in long term treatment of gout can be good. But, there are risks as well as little evidence. Uricosuric drugs could worsen an existing condition such as gout. Because acute inflammation can be treated with other medication, some doctors prefer to wait until a month before recommending uricosuric treatment. Uricosurics, such as "probenecid", could increase the severity of acute attacks but not prevent them. In order to lessen the initial gout attack-inducing effect that uricosurics can have, colchicine and probenecid are sometimes combined.

Contraindications. In general, these drugs shouldn't be taken if there is a risk of developing a bladder infection or stones, or if the patient is undergoing chemotherapy or radiation for cancer. Patients over 60 are generally advised not to use drugs such as probenecid. It is not recommended to take probenecid if you are also taking aspirin. You should exercise caution if your family has a history of peptic.

Side effects: Probenecid/sulfinpyrazone could cause skin rashes and kidney stone formation. You can prevent kidney stones from forming by drinking enough water and reducing your caffeine intake. Supplementation with sodium bicarbonate can also help to reduce acidity.

Interactions with other drugs. Because probenecid or uricosurics lowers the kidneys' ability to remove antibiotics from the body it is sometimes used in combination with penicillin to increase blood levels of the antibiotic. Probenecid and other uricosuric drugs may interact with hypertension drug

(ACE-inhibitors such as captopril), NSAIDs such indometacin or ketoprofen (ibuprofen/ibuprofen), certain antimetabolite/antifolate drugs(methotrexate), and certain "water pills/loop uric drugs (furosomide), antibiotics and penicillins (G, V, procaine and benzathine), AZT medicines, ganciclovir ganciclovir/acyclovir

Aspirin, when taken in low doses is considered to be an anti-uricosuric medicine. Aspirin can raise blood levels and decrease urine levels of the uric Acid. The effects of uricosuric drugs will be countered if you take aspirin (acetylsalicylic acids or asa), in low doses.

Probenecid and other drugs that urosurics can interfere with some laboratory tests such as the glucose test.

Inhibitors of Xanthine Oxidase

Xanthine oxidase, also known as XO, is an enzyme responsible for purine metabolism.

Uric acid levels in the blood can be reduced by blocking this enzyme. The XO inhibitor medications can be divided into two categories: purine analogues or "others". Analogues to purine include allopurinol (Zyloprim), Zyloric, and oxypurinol (which are the active metabolites of allopurinol). Apart from the analogues we also find (making up "other" xanthine oxide inhibitors), febuxostat ("Uloric"), topiroxostat [Topiloric], Uriadec] and inositols. Although it was once considered part of the vitamin B Complex, it is not an essential nutritional element per definition since it is produced by our bodies from glucose.

XO-inhibitors are often used for patients who cannot or won't be able to take uricosuric medicines due to kidney problems. XOs-inhibitors, specifically allopurinol are a key component of the treatment and prevention of gout. There have been many brands such as Zyloprim, Zyloric, and Zyloric. Febuxostat (Uloric), a newer XO inhibiting drug, has been shown to be more effective than allopurinol in some studies. In two clinical trials, febuxostat treated patients reached the primary end point significantly faster than allopurinol. In the subset with impaired kidney function, Febuxostat was superior to allopurinol. Mild-to-moderate impairment does not require dose adjustment. Long-term extension trials confirmed the efficacy, and tolerance of febuxostat. Patients who achieved the target level of 6 mg/dl (360 Mmol/l) saw a steady decline in the number of gout flares. Many of the patients experienced tophi resolution. Similar to allopurinol, febuxostat caused nausea, dizziness diarrhoea and headaches.

Effectiveness: Gout attacks are usually prevented by XO-inhibitors. Allopurinol is listed on the WHO's List of Essential Medicines. For the medication to work fully, it must be taken for at least 2 to 3 months. In a persistent gout attack, allopurinol could worsen the condition or even trigger it. XO-inhibitors may also be prescribed as colchicine, NSAIDs, and for a time (usually a few month) after an attack.

Contraindications, interactions, warnings : Pregnancy. Patients taking medications such azathioprine (mercaptopurine), or theophylline. Patients suffering from liver disease should undergo periodic liver function testing during the early stages of treatment. Gout flares are possible during the first months of therapy. Patients with diminished renal function will need to take lower doses. Ask your doctor to discuss the drugs n this particular group.

Side effects: It is possible to get rashes, fever, or hepatitis from taking XO-inhibitors, such as allopurinol. Allopurinol may cause several life-threatening dermatological problems. Although rare, it may occur. Hypersensitivity can occur with any drug. It is important to be aware of the symptoms and quickly react to them if they present. Some people may have mild skin reactions, but they can adapt to allopurinol. Allopurinol might also cause cataracts, leucopenia, and thrombocytopenia. Allopurinol could also have a side effect that lowers blood pressure. This may make it a good choice for patients with hypertension or gout. Febuxostat may cause nausea and rash as well as a reduced liver function.

Mitotic Inhibitors

Colchicine is used for both acute and chronic gout. Find out more about colchicine by clicking here.

Newer drugs

Gout was once considered an obscure disease. Even worse, the US market was only worth 50 million US dollar per year. This meant that pharmaceutical companies were not interested in investing much money or time in it. The rise in gout patients has made this situation change. The potential goldmine for drug companies is here. One of the positive aspects is that many new drugs have been developed and are currently being put on the market. Canakinumab ("Ilaris") has been mentioned as an alternative to NSAIDs.

Chapter 15: Dietary Problems (Foods Not To Eat, Foods Not To Eat)

Gout has been associated for a long time with diet, in particular overindulgence or gluttony. It is often called the "death of the kings." Gout was an affliction that Henry the VIII, the English monarch, suffered from. Susanne's "At The King's Table" book reveals that Henry VIII was served a fast meal of soup, cod (pike, cod), lampreys, pike and salmon in 1526. This was just the beginning.

What foods can cause gout?

Gout is usually seen in people with gout. However, there are many foods that "trigger" the condition. Some people have difficulty eating spinach, while others can't eat it. There are many triggers.

All sufferers of gout "know" they must avoid purine rich foods. Purine is concentrated most often in foods like oysters. But do you eat a lot more liver and kidney than normal? Do you regularly eat brains? Ox hearts or sweetbreads? You could also add a few smokedherrings to your daily lunches of mackerel, wild game, elk, and deer. Nc? Are you still suffering from gout? Do you think a low purine diet is the best thing for most gout sufferers or not?

If purine were not the problem, then gout would be much less of a problem since most people don't eat high levels of purine foods. Gout is a problem. It is actually on the rise. Gout cases have more than doubled in the UK over the past decade. Are they eating too many liver and sardines suddenly? Steak and kidney pie are two of the most popular English dishes. However, there has been a decline in the popularity of these traditional dishes. The consumption of beer has also declined as younger consumers are more inclined to drink spirits, while many more people are turning their attention to wine. This notion that diet plays an important part in our health makes sense. Not so if you think about the purine rich foods. Gout can also be caused by uric and uric acid excretion. So what can a person suffering from gout do?

Myths and Facts on Foods to Avoid

Because uric acids levels need to be decreased, doctors emphasize the fact that purine rich foods should be avoided. You will need to avoid eating foods that are high in purines. Sardines in oil (480mg. Uric acid per 100g), ox live (555 mg.), chicken liver (554mg.), and pig's liver (515mg.), sweetbread for calf (1260mg.), baker's yeast (680mg.), and smoked sprat (804mg.). are all prohibited. An unsmoked sprat is, apparently, acceptable. It doesn't really matter to us, as I don't know what a "sprat" is. It is possible to reduce the intake of purine rich foods but it won't make a difference in reducing your risk of developing gout attacks. You should forget purines being the main cause of gout. This is the one and only group of "purines" that can cause gout.

There are several types of purines

Purines are amino acid building blocks of proteins. There are many kinds of purines. In simple words, purines contain a base as well as ribose or deoxyribose and also phosphoric. The most important purine bases include adenine and guanine as well as hypoxanthine, xanthine, xanthine, xanthine and hypoxanthine. Research has shown that hypoxanthine (xanthine) and xanthine are purines that are most likely increase uric Acid levels. While adenine, guanine and other purines based on guanine may be safer. The ethanol makes the Guanine more dangerous for people with gout, possibly excepting beer. According to other studies, purines made from plants are less harmful than those from animals. Additionally, purines made from milk are less harmful than other purines.

Purifications for animals

Yuqing Zhang at Boston University did an interesting study and found that purine from animals poses a greater risk of causing a Gout Attack than purine obtained from plants. In addition to showing that purine consumption can lead to gout attacks and that purines from plant sources are more dangerous than purine from animals, the study also shows that purines found in foods made from purines of plants are less harmful to your health. This study also shows that a high intake of purines in short-term meals can produce flares as well as a high level of purines in a regular diet.

To find out when and what 633 gout sufferers ate before their flare ups, the study followed them. The median purine intake in 2-day control periods was 0.06 Oz. the equivalent of about 3.1 pounds for men. 64.1 lb. You can also eat spinach. In the two days preceding a gout flare men ate on average 0.07 oz. A purine would have weighed in at 3.8 lbs. 7 lbs. of beef You can also eat spinach. Researchers found that purine intakes from animals were five times higher than those from plant foods, with 0.03 oz. versus 0.006 oz. Over a 2-day span. Zhang and co-workers observed, "Our findings support that plant-derived food should be the preferred source for protein for gout sufferers, since they are excellent sources of fiber, vitamins, minerals, and have also been studied against the risk factors of weight gain and sudden cardiac deaths.

Some foods have high purine content

A table containing some foods and their purine content is enclosed to help you understand which foods contain high amounts of purines. Data taken from Kiyoko Kanno's study "Total and Purine Base content of Common Foodstuffs to Facilitate Nutritional Therapy for Gout & Hyperuricemia", 2014. Gout sufferers shouldn't eat foods that are high in purines or very high in them.

Very High

More than 300 mg in 100 grams

Chlorella 3182,7

Beer yeast 2995.7

Dried anchovy 1108,6

Spirulina 1086,8

Nori 591,70

Dried Shiitake mushroom 379.50

High

200 to 300mg per 100g

Monkfish liver, steamed 399,20

Sardine, 305.70

Parsley 288,90

Liver from pork 284,80

Liver from beef 219.80

Moderate

100 to 200mg per 100g

Beef kidney 174,20

Soybean, dried, 172.50

Spinach,young leaf 171,80

Tuna,fresh 157,40

Crab 152.20

Clam 145.50

Beef, topside 143.50

Chicken breast 141.20

Herring 139.60

Chicken wing 137,50

Parma ham 138.30

Octopus, 137.30

Sea urchin 137.30

Oyster sauce 134,40

Broccoli sprouts 129.60

Chicken leg 122,90

Salami 120.40

Chicken skin 119,70

Pork tenderloin 119,70

Salmon, fresh 119.30

Fermented soybean,Natto 113,90

Pork Rump 113,000.

Whale meat

Whale meat 111.30

Pork shoulder/knee, 107.60

Beef shin: 106,40

Spiny lobster, 102,10

Rice Bran 100,2

Low

50 to 100mg per 100g

Beef, tenderloin 98,40

Caviar 94,70

Pork, sirloin 90,90

Beef, shoulder sirloin, 90,20

Pork shoulder 81.40

Beef, brisket: 79.20

Beef, shoulder and ribs 77.40

Buckwheat flour 75.90

Pork, ribs 75.80

Boneless Ham 74.20

Beef, ribloin 74,20

White raddish sprigs 73.20

Pork neck 70.50

Monkfish 70,00

Green pepper 69.20

Red miso 63,50

Bacon 61,80

Squid: 59,60

Cauliflower 57.20

Japanese pumpkin 56.60

Asparagus 55.30

Deep-fried Tofu 54.40

Spinach 51,40

Eggplant 50.70

Very Low

There are less than 50 mg in 100 grams

Frankfurt sausage 49,80

Peanut 49.10

Corned Beef 47,00

Vienna sausage 45,50

Soy sauce,dark 45,20

Broad bean 35.50

Almond 31,40

Rice 25,90

Flor, bread 25,80

Soy milk 22,00

Herring roe 21,90

Ramen noodle 21,60

Avocado 18,40

Garlic 17,00

Salmon roe 15,70

Deep fried rice cracker 14,10

Corn 11,70

Asparagus Lower Part 10,20

Cucumber 9,40

Yoghurt 5,20

Cabbage 3,20

Banana 3,00

Carrot 2,20

Strawberry 2,10

Chicken egg 0,00

Milk 0,00

Click here to see data source

Avoid fructose

Everyday, more people are speaking out about the dangers that fructose can cause. Fructose (sugar) is all around us. Americans consume around 200 pounds of sugar annually. This was 4.100 years ago. Yes, we did go from four to 200lbs sugar in three generations. You think this has had some negative consequences. Many believe that sugar alone is responsible not only for obesity, diabetes, but also for other health issues such as gout.

Sugar comes under many names and forms. All depend on the source of sugar. Sacchar is the Greek word for sugar. There are simple sugars and complex sugars. Monosaccharide refers to simple sugars. This literally means "single Sugar". Fructose can be described as a simple sugar or monosaccharide. Also, glucose and galactose are both single sugars. These simple sugars are the building blocks for complex sugars like disaccharids, Oligosaccahrids or Polysacchards. Two monosaccharids compose diasaccharids. Oligosaccharides can have three to nine. Polysaccharids can have many more.

There are also sucrose, lactose and other simple sugars. When you hear sugar, most people think of crystallized white table syrup, which is better known as sucrose. Sucrose can be described as a mixture of simple sugars fructose or glucose.

Sugars are carbohydrates. Simple sugars, simple carbohydrates, are quick energy. This means that the energy is consumed quickly. The effects are felt immediately, but you also lose them quickly. Powerful, but quick. Complex sugars, or complex carbohydrates, can often be linked to fiber. They are slower carbohydrates. Table sugar is the bond between fructose or glucose. Sucrose may be thought to be healthier because it is more complex than a simple sweetener, but fructose helps in fructose's absorption.

Doctor Hyon Choi is an individual who has made many important and potentially groundbreaking studies about gout. He has studied the link between fructose consumption and gout. According to one of his studies, people who consume sugary soft drink have an increased chance of developing gout. Sweetened drinks are more at risk. Choi found that gout attacks were more common in men who drink five to six soft beverages per week than in those who consume one drink per monthly. The likelihood of getting gout from drinking two soft drinks per week was 85% higher for those who drank more than one drink per month. Choi also concluded that diet soft drink consumption is not associated with gout. Choi also noted that the same applies to fruit juices, which are equally linked to the risk of gout attack and gout. What is the common ingredient of diet soft drinks? Fructose.

Gout can be caused when you eat too much fructose

Numerous studies show that fructose has been linked to gout. A diet high in fructose may cause or worsen gout. This is a common explanation for the recent rise in gout symptoms. It also removes the outdated notion that a gout patient is a gourmet or gourmand who eats calf, liver, brains, lobsters, and you'll be fine if your diet stops consuming purine rich food. It is clear that the list of foods you must avoid is much longer and more complicated. Certain foods are more crucial to avoid than others.

Fructose can be linked to gout. It is linked to many other health conditions, conditions, syndromes, diseases such as elevated LDL cholesterol or triglycerides.

High-fructose corn Syrup

Fructose, a commonly used additive in factory-produced food and drinks, is very common. If you think about Coke, or any other sugary fizz drinks, then you will see a rich source for fructose. It is thanks to high-fructose, corn syrup, one of the most important additives in food today. Producers of this cheap sweetener take corn syrups, and then expose them to enzymes to extract more glucose. The result is more sweetened. 55, which is 55% fructose/42% glucose, is the most common corn syrup found in soft drinks. The rest is water.

The truth is that Coca-Cola uses even more fructose - up to 65 percent. High-fructose Corn Syrup is preferred to sucrose by large companies. This is because it's more affordable to produce and because it has a special sweetness that can be addictive. The US government would prefer to use US-grown corn rather than imported sugarcane. The government does not just want to promote US corn, but also imposes additional taxes or tariffs upon imported sucrose. All this is done to protect the US corn farmer. In the US, sucrose is more expensive than anywhere else. One curious side note is that Coca Cola enthusiasts love Brazilian or Mexican Coca Cola. This is because it's sweetened not with high-fructose syrup. They like it better with sucrose.

Is it okay to consume glucose?

It's back to gout. Because fructose, if it is bad, high-fructose syrup from corn syrup is even worse. Avoid corn syrup-sweetened soft drinks. What about soft drinks that are sweetened with sucrose Can sucrose be considered a complex sugar and more than just a simple sugar. It is possible that it could be healthier and safe for people with gout to consume. While it is possible that sucrose could be "healthier" than high glucose corn syrup, this doesn't necessarily mean it is better. In relation to fructose (which is known to be dangerous for those suffering from gout), sucrose actually allows fructose to potentially be uptaken by glucose when it appears to be bound to fructose. What about glucose as a whole? You won't notice an increase in uric Acid levels if you consume pure glucose. Studies have again shown that glucose is healthier than monosaccharides and is therefore a healthier sugar. Glucose could be used as a food sweetener to treat gout. Only when glucose is made readily available for sweetening purposes will we be able really to tell. You can buy it, even though it isn't in all supermarkets. It's not a good idea to sweeten fruit juices or other sweetened foods with natural fructose. Reducing the use of high-fructose Corn Syrup.

Avoid fruits

However, it is not necessary to point the finger at sugary beverages. Fruits contain a lot of fructose. Yes. Fruits are more than good for you. This may surprise you but it is the only conclusion you can reach from looking at the facts. Did you think gout was only about avoiding beer and lobster? Soft drinks should not be your enemy. Fruit juices deserve more respect. Juicing involves removing the pulp from the fruits, which can lead to a loss of fiber. Are you concerned about gout developing or worsening? Get a high-fructose apple juice, remove the pulp, and add sucrose. Although eating fruit is healthier, it's best for those with gout.

Can you eat all fruits?

Some fruits are higher in fructose than other. Bananas, bananas (including strawberries), avocados, lemons, and limes) are moderate to low-fructose. Fruits such as grapes, pears, apples and grapes contain high levels of fructose. Vegetables, too, contains fructose. Asparagus, leafy greens and spinach are among the vegetables that have moderate to low levels. Fruit is not allowed in meat, but dairy products that are lactose-free are acceptable.

You should remember that processed foods contain high levels of sugars, fructose and other sweeteners. Some breakfast cereals may contain up to 40% sugar by weight. As such, cereal bars are not recommended for people with gout. Ice cream and cakes contain sugar. So are many other condiments, dressings, or sauces. Raspberry vinaigrette contains a lot sugar. Ketchup is not the only culprit. If you enjoy alcohol, avoid brandy and other liquors. Cooler wine is not the best option, so avoid energy drinks like Frappuccino and brandy. Because of the fruit's fructose, unsweetened fruit juice might be harmful for gout sufferers. Unsweetened apple liquid is the same as soda.

Plan a gout-friendly diet. This is a diet that reduces the likelihood of gout attacks. The main concern is the uric level. To manage your gout, it is important to avoid high levels. Purine is a well-known factor. While this may be true, it is important to keep in mind a few points, such as the fact that purines are not all equal. Fructose is a likely factor in gout and should be reduced.

Some fruits have high fructose levels

Food Fructose gr/100g

Dates 32.00

Raisins 29.70

Dryed figs 22,90

Prunes 12.50

Grapes 8.13

Pears 6.23

Cherries 6.00

Apples 5.90

Blueberry 4.97

Bananas 4.85

Kiwi 4.35

Watermelon 3.36

Plums 3.07

Honeydew melon 2.96

Grapefruit 2.50

Strawberry 2.50

Blackberry 2.40

Raspberry 2.35

Orange 2.25

Pineapple 2.05

Cantaloupe 1.87

Peach 1.53

Nectarine 1.37

Apricot 0.94

Data taken directly from this site.

Carbohydrates & Insulin Resistance Syndrome

There are studies that show that not only is purine, in particular from animal protein, bad for gout sufferers but that cutting down on all carbohydrate intake could significantly reduce the likelihood of gout flare-ups. Dr. P. H. Dessein conducted research that found that gout flares in a group with a history of gout attacks decreased when they were given a low-carbohydrate meal of 160 grams per day. The diet included 1600 calories per daily with 40% coming from carbohydrates and 30% from proteins. This diet had a remarkable 2 mg./dl decrease in uric Acid. These results indicate that the uric acids lowering effects of decreasing carbohydrate intake for gout patients was much better than other protein-diminishing foods.

These results are important for understanding how to best manage your weight. Foods that have a low purine content tend to be high-in saturated fat and carbohydrates. You should not give low-purine diet advice.

Iron rich food

Studies have shown that too much iron could be a problem for those suffering from gout. Many studies have shown that high levels iron (or ferritin), are often associated with high levels uric Acid. Francesco S. Facchini, 2003, shows that gout patients who are hyperuric acidic have their symptoms improve when iron levels are reduced. F. S. Facchini led the research and removed iron from 12 patients in order to get the lowest amount of iron possible without making them anemic. These results revealed that gouty attacks had decreased.

Iron-rich foods include meats, pork, seafood, eggs, beans, spinach, and – surprisingly - any processed food which has iron. This is quite a lot of food these days. It's worth noting, however, that many of traditional gouty foods such as seafood, livers, oysters, musses, and clams have the highest levels of iron per kilogram. Liver comes in at number two. Even if pumpkin seeds don't get eaten a lot, you may find it interesting to learn that they are a good three-source of iron. Avoid eating most types of nuts. The next step is meats. To give an idea of iron content, oysters have 28 mg. per 100 grams. Liver is around 23 mg. Pumpkin seed has 15 mg. while nuts contain 6 mg. The iron in lean tenderloins of beef drops to approximately 3 mg per 100 grams, making it more moderate than oysters.

Do not eat breakfast cereals enriched in iron, regardless of what you do.

Some foods have high iron content

FOODMG PER 100 GRAMS

Kellogg's All Bran Compleat 62,10

Cheerios, cereal 33,17

Kellogs Corn Flakes 28,90

Liver, pork raw 23,3

White beans, raw 10,44

Liver,beef 844

Parsley fresh 6,20

Liver,beef pan-fried 6,17

Goose liver pate 5,50

Black beans, raw 5,02

Quinoa,uncooked 4,57

Squash and pumpkin seed 3,31

Egg yolk,raw 2,73

Spinach,raw 2,71

Beef, tenderloin raw 2,18

Egg,whole raw 1,75

Mollusks,clams raw 1,62

Lamb,tenderloin 1,62

Pork tenderloin and pork, raw 0,97

Chicken breast, raw w/skin 0,74

Fish Cod, raw 0,38

Egg white, 0,08

Data taken directly from here.

Alcohol intake

Gout symptoms can be greatly reduced by reducing alcohol intake for those who drink and have gout problems. Kiyoko Kaneko (a Japanese scientist) has attempted to determine the purine content of different types of alcohol. His 1985 study revealed greater differences than was previously thought. Beer is worse then other drinks, while high-malt beverages are the worst. Although it isn't known exactly which brand or type, whisky had significantly lower levels of purines than alcohol. For an example, beer had a purine count between 4-6 mg. per Liter, while whisky was 0.12 mg. The purine content of Japanese beer is much lower than imported beer. In 2010, Dr. Jae Bu Jun and the Korean Rheumatism Association performed a similar study. Beer contained significantly more purines in beer than distilled beverages.

Theobromine

Gout sufferers with gout will be interested in theobromine. If you examine tables listing purine-rich foods, you'll see that it has a very high rating. It contains 2300mg. purires for each 100 grams. Theobromine/xantheose is a bitter alkaloid of the cacao plant. It can be found in cocoa and chocolate as well tea. Theobromine in its pure form is toxic. Cacao, chocolate, and chocolate both conta n low amounts of theobromine that make them safe for human intake. But is it safe to gout sufferers? Some even advocate using theobromine to stop gout attacks. What is the point of using theobromine as a high-purine food?

In fact, theobromine has many uses. It lowers blood tension. It works as a vasodilator thanks to the flavanols ([3]) it contains. Numerous studies suggest that flavanols might provide significant vascular defense due to their antioxidant capabilities and increased nitric dioxide bioavailability. Nitric oxide bioavailability, in turn, has a significant impact on insulin-stimulated diabetes uptake as well as vascular tone. Flavanols might also have beneficial metabolic and pressor effects. It may be useful in asthma treatment and it can also help to ease cough. There are some negative side effects, however, such as a study that found an association between theobromine use and prostate cancer. Side note: Dog owners should know that chocolate may be fatal for dogs due to the high level of theobromine in it. Dogs don't metabolize chocolate as fast, so even 50 grams of dark chocolate can poison a small dog.

Now, back to gout. Gout sufferers may not feel the effects of theobromine's purine level because it is a plant-based drug. Flavonols might be another reason it's worth taking theobromine.

Myths about foods to eat

This leads us to the next section, where we'll be discussing foods that may help to control gout. Let's start at the beginning.

Dehydration

Water is a very basic and simple aspect of diet. People search for miracle pills or super-foods which may mysteriously or powerfully combat a disease. The reality is usually more complex and saddening. Gout is no exception. However, water might be an effective "drug" for gout.

To say water is important would be an understatement. Water is the basis of all living things. Although you can live several weeks without food and water, it is enough to kill you in a matter of days. It is such an ingredient, so fundamental to human existence, we don't even consider water an important ingredient. Water is essential to human health. Gout sufferers in particular may drink too little. Gout can be triggered by dehydration, according to many doctors. "Defhydration can lead to an increase in serum uric Acid levels. It can also decrease the kidney's capacity to remove uric Acid and increase the risk of crystal formation. All of these factors together can increase the likelihood of having gout attack. Tuhina Neogi MD and PhD, the lead author of a Boston University School of Medicine research, said that water can reverse the dehydration effects. This study was presented at Philadelphia's 2009 American College of Rheumatology annual meeting. It showed that drinking between five and eight glasses of water per daily reduced the chance of suffering from gout attacks by an astounding 40%. In fact, the study found that the less water a gout patient consumes, the less likely he has an attack.

It's not easy to drink enough water, as we all know. This is a simple way to relieve gout. Keep hydrated. Keep hydrated. Although 8 cups of water is the standard, it is not recommended to do so every day. This "tip" comes from a 1945 Food and Nutrition Board campaign that was poorly understood. IOM doesn't provide any tips on water intake these days, but it does give us an indication of thirst. IOM recommended 16 cups of "total fluid" for men (approximately 3.75 liters) while women should consume 11.5 cups (approximately 2.75 liters). You should remember that water intakes do not solely depend on actual water. It also includes fluids (foods that contain water). Keep in mind that the same sources advise men to drink 3 liters per daily of total drinks (13 cups) while women need 2.2liters (9 cups).

Gout sufferers may find relief in coffee, as we'll see. Keep in mind, however, that coffee will not help you if you don't drink enough water.

Coffee and chocolate (or xanthine)

A happy pairing of food: chocolate and coffee. It is not a coincidence that most of the drinks we drink contain caffeine and chocolate. Many scientists would agree. They believe that methylxanthine has the ability to make chocolate and coffee more delicious. Methylxanthine can be described as a methylated form of xanthine. Two compounds of chocolate and coffee are caffeine and theobromine. Other methylxanthines included theophylline. Aminopfylline. Paraxanthine. Pentoxfylline. Pentoxfylline treats muscle pain due to early-stage peripheral arterial disease. Drugs such as aminofylline, theophylline, and aminofylline can be used for various airway conditions. Two compounds within a group are caffeine and theobromine. They should be considered drugs. They are powerful drugs. All drugs are derived xanthines (or purines).

Why then, is purine bad for gout sufferers when purines can be a helpful supplement? All purines aren't created equal, as we know. You must distinguish between animal- and plant-based purines. Purines should not be viewed as one homogenous group that does nothing but increase uric Acid levels.

Theobromine, caffeine, and theobromine are two of the most prominent methylxanthines contained in cacao. Because of their remarkable health benefits, chocolate is often considered a functional foods. Flavanols, which are an important component of cocoa, have a lot of antioxidant properties. Perhaps the anti-inflammatory properties of flavanols from chocolate and coffee are due to their role in chocolate. Epicatechins, in particular, are a key ingredient in cocoa. The mechanisms of all these compounds are still unknown and complex. While there is very little information about this, evidence is increasing. If you're looking for first-line intelligence on how to treat gout, chocolate and coffee are two options. There are several studies, including a 12-year study with over 45,000 males. H. K. Choi, a gout researcher concluded that long-term coffee use is associated with a lower likelihood of developing incident gout. A new study (Felix Grases 2014) has concluded that theobromine can inhibit nucleation or crystal growth of uric and that it may be clinically helpful in the treatment of uric nephrolithiasis.

Low-fat dairy product

Studies have shown that there is an inverse correlation between low-fat milk intake and gout risk (Nicola Dalbeth 2010). A separate study, also conducted by Nicola Dalbeth revealed that skimmed milk powder enriched w/ glycomacropeptides/G600 milk fat extract significantly reduced gout flares in gout sufferers, as well as big improvements in pain and stiffness. Cow's Milk may have an anti-inflammatory and acute urate-lowering effects. It was also found that those who consumed one cup of milk daily over a period of six years in an American study with 15,000 people showed a significant reduction in their levels of uric Acid. Clear benefits were also seen in cheese-lovers.

Vitamin C

Vitamin C may help to excrete uric Acid, according to some theories. There are some indications that vitamin C may help lower the production of Uric acid. However, a new study by Lisa Stamp of the University of Otago in Christchurch New Zealand found that vitamin

C didn't lower the levels of uric Acid in gout patients.

Summary Dietary Tips/A way Forward

Let's now sum up all this diet information. Be sure to consult your doctor before you begin to implement any diet tips. Also, the following tips do not include medication and are strictly diet tips.

Before you change your diet, make sure you take into consideration all medications that you are on as well as any other medical conditions.

First, moderation seems to be the key. It may be necessary to take some drastic measures to maintain a moderate lifestyle in the future. Reduce the amount of food and drinks you eat, or drink. It is difficult to maintain moderation, especially when you consider that you might have gout. It is best to do so for a short time. While this doesn't mean that you should not enjoy some of the foods mentioned above, it does suggest that moderation is important. While I do not know your diet, it is possible that you are already using some or all of these tips. Controlling gout isn't about avoiding certain foods or ingredients. It's about managing your entire diet.

Massive changes

My suggestion is to cut down on certain foods for 30 day and then come back to reevaluate the situation. Be aware that your doctor will need to review any dietary changes you make before you can implement them.

* Get rid of all sugary fizzy drinks, including fructose.

* Get rid of all fruit juices that contain added sugar (fructose/other sugars).

* Avoid sweetened yoghurts (but don't eliminate yoghurts) (fructose or other sugars).

* Stop eating fast food (fructose, sugars, iron additions).

* Eliminate all alcohol (because it has an all-round effect on gout).

* Eliminate the use of table sugar.

* Eliminate all candy, even chocolate bars.

* Get rid of all processed foods, such as breads, cereals, and soups.

* Remove all red meat, pork or lamb, as well as seafood (iron/purine content).

* No nuts, seeds or pumkin seed. It is possible to eat pumpkin.

* Take out spinach and beans to reduce iron content

* Eliminate spirulina (purine)

* Eliminate sardines, anchovies (purine contents).

* Take out the parsley (purine & iron content).

You might be wondering: what is the best way to eat chicken? First of all, chicken is safe to eat in moderation. You can eat eggs. Tofu. You can eat legumes such as eggplant. Green salads are allowed, but not the spinach. You can eat onions and radishes as well as celery. Potatoes. Moderation is key with pasta and ramen noodles. Cauliflowers such as asparagus, peas, and mushroom are not okay. But you should eat white fish, such as monkfish, and, if they are more readily available, cod and salmon. Seaweed is best avoided when eating sushi. You should eat less fruit. If you are a smoothie and fruit juice fan, reduce the amount of fruit juices. You should eat no more than 1-2 fruits per day, both pulp and whole. Garlic is great anti-inflammatory agent. You can use fresh rosemary with your weekly chicken dinner.

This detox is intended to increase awareness, particularly regarding processed foods and sugar. You must register any changes made to the menu items you are adding back. Check out how it feels. As a guide, use the purine, fructose, and iron-lists, but be open for other foods that may cause gout. It is important to remember that your detox does not mean you should avoid all foods that can trigger gout. Instead, your goal is to reduce certain foods, and to gain a better understanding of your own triggers.

Food diary

It might be worthwhile to keep a food log. Keep track of everything you eat. Then, if you experience a flare-up in your gout, you can refer to your food diary to find out what you ate the previous weeks. You might try taking photos with your smartphone of what you have eaten. Get a uric acid meter kit and test your levels frequently, maybe even every week. To truly understand your gout and to reduce your chance of new flare-ups, you can do tests every day. Every person is unique, so it will help you find what works for you.

After the 30-day period, reevaluate the list. Red meat should not be included in your diet. Moderation is key. Breakfast cereals, soft drinks, commercial fruit juices and other beverages are likely to be unhealthy. You can decide. Try it out.

This "gout detox" for 30 days will give you the foundation you need to add food in moderation.

To add to the list below, you can also reduce your intake of certain foods during your 30-day detox. However, this should not be your only option.

* Carbohydrates

Apart from removing certain foods entirely and decreasing carbs, you should also add other foods.

Drink at least 3 Liters of water per day if a man and 2 Liters if a woman.

www.ingramcontent.com/pod-product-compliance
Lightning Source LLC
Chambersburg PA
CBHW060500030426
42337CB00015B/1671